Medicine and Literature

The doctor's companion to the classics

John Salinsky

Foreword by
Iona Heath CBE

Radcliffe Medical Press

Radcliffe Medical Press Ltd
18 Marcham Road
Abingdon
Oxon OX14 1AA
United Kingdom

www.radcliffe-oxford.com
The Radcliffe Medical Press electronic catalogue and online ordering facility.
Direct sales to anywhere in the world.

British Library Cataloguing in Publication Data

A catalogue record for this book is available from the British Library.

ISBN 1 85775 535 9

Typeset by Advance Typesetting Ltd, Oxfordshire
Printed and bound by TJ International Ltd, Padstow, Cornwall

Contents

Foreword

In different ways, novelists, doctors and patients all seek to understand and express what it is to be human. Patients come to doctors to give an account of experience and sensations that they have found troubling or difficult. They must find words to communicate their distress and the listening doctor must find words to signal that he or she has at least partly understood. Novelists use words in ways which show that they have understood parts of the experience of all of us. We find incidents in the stories of fictional characters which resonate exactly with the reality of our lives, and the expressive ability of the writer gives new dimensions to our own experience. We begin to think about our patients and ourselves in a different, deeper way, and all our interactions are the richer.

Too many years ago, as a very young GP principal, I was invited to join an established Balint group. It was there that I first encountered John Salinsky and his boundless and infectious enthusiasm for human stories. Then it was the stories told by his patients; now, in this book, he brings the same qualities to the stories of literature.

In 1989, I applied for extended study leave and was summoned for an interview at the Department of Postgraduate Education. Our practice had agreed that each partner should have a three-month sabbatical every 10 years. Our children were at school and travel was not an option, and so, for three months, my plan was to sit on the sofa and read novels. At that time, medical humanities had yet to emerge as a legitimate academic endeavour and my proposed programme seemed to be regarded as frivolous by those who held the purse strings. My application was turned down. I went ahead anyway and those three marvellous months had the most profoundly revitalising effect on my perception of my patients and of what it is to be a doctor. I rediscovered my childhood joy in reading, which had been submerged by the pressures of study and work. My original plan had been to read novels in the mornings and to be a perfect mother in the afternoons. I had visions of my children arriving home from school not as latchkey kids, but to the smell of fresh baking and the whirr of the sewing machine. But all this went by the board as I found myself completely unable to tear myself away from my reading, so that I stopped only when they were clamouring for supper. I had chosen the novels with care, writing to a panel of friends to ask which 10 books they would read if they were allowed only 10 in a lifetime. There was a quite remarkable consistency in the first five or six choices and, to my shame, I had read almost none of them. Three of them – *Bleak House*, *Anna Karenin* and *Middlemarch* – are on John Salinsky's list.

I still haven't read all the books that John and his co-authors recommend, but their enthusiasm is irresistible and, having read this book, I know that I must. I will start with *Tristram Shandy*.

Iona Heath
July 2001

About the authors

John Salinsky is a General Practitioner in Wembley, Middlesex, and Course Organiser at the Whittington Vocational Training Scheme for General Practice. Since 1998 he has been responsible for the 'Medicine and Literature' column in the journal *Education for Primary Care* (formerly *Education for General Practice*).

Brian Glasser is Honorary Lecturer at the Royal Free Hospital, London, in the Department of Population Science and Primary Care, where he teaches medical sociology and communications skills.

Gillie Bolton is Research Fellow in Medical Humanities at Sheffield University Institute of General Practice.

Oliver Samuel was for many years a General Practitioner in Pinner, Middlesex, and Vocational Training Course Organiser at Northwick Park Hospital, Harrow. He has recently retired from his post as Lecturer at the University of Westminster.

Alistair Stead is Senior Fellow in English Literature at the University of Leeds.

Tim Swanwick is a General Practitioner in Watford, Herts, and Deputy Dean in the Department of General Practice at Thames Postgraduate Medical and Dental Education.

1

Introduction: why should doctors read the classics?

When I was at school, my best subjects were English and biology. Biology taught me how living things worked, which interested me greatly because l knew it was the first step on the path to becoming a doctor. But, as the narrow sixth form science curriculum began to close around me, I had some regrets that I would no longer be able to learn more about literature – except in my own time and without any help from teachers.

During my years at medical school and as a hospital doctor, the prescribed reading was all firmly focused on biological and clinical science. Nevertheless, I continued reading for pleasure and extending my knowledge of the classics. Some of them I found difficult and perplexing, but with many there was an immediate spark of connection, as if the author was speaking to me directly and we understood each other perfectly. These books gave me great enjoyment and the sense that I had discovered hidden treasure. Their stories were always there for me to revisit and the characters took up residence in my inner world.

When I became a family doctor, I found myself in a world where people were constantly telling me their stories and sharing their feelings with me. Often they reminded me of people in my favourite books, and the fictional characters I read about would remind me of particular patients I had encountered, so that the two worlds would reflect each other. And they still do. A young woman, hopelessly in love with the wrong man will remind me of Anna Karenin; a frightened, anorexic little waif makes me think of Fanny Price from *Mansfield Park*; a clever but tormented student could be Joyce's Stephen Dedalus; and the family of three brothers in my practice, of whom the elder two are schizophrenic, always make me think of the Karamazov boys.

Lines and phrases from literature also float into my mind as I listen to the patients: 'All happy families are alike: but every unhappy family is unhappy in its own way' – that one comes up a lot. An angry man, incoherently vowing vengeance, conjures up: 'I shall do such things, I know not yet what they be, but they shall be as the terrors of the earth' (from *King Lear*). Someone expressing anguished regret makes me think: 'agenbite of inwit' (James Joyce's wonderful borrowed but freshly applied phrase for the gnawing of conscience). And, when an amiable old fellow launches himself on an apparently pointless digression (as they frequently do), I remember Tristram Shandy declaring that 'digressions are incontestably the sunshine'. That always helps me to sit back and listen and not worry about the diagnosis, which will come at its own appointed time.

Has all this awareness of literary parallels in the consulting room helped me to be a better doctor? That would be hard to prove. It certainly helps me to see my patients as human beings. And because they resemble my old friends, the characters in my favourite books, I think I am able to regard at least some of them in a more benign, forgiving and tolerant way. I become less impatient with them and more interested in their feelings. I feel sure that there are times when thinking about the classics has helped me to be amused rather than enraged when patients behave in ways which doctors traditionally hate. I am thinking of the 'trivial complaints', the 'inappropriate demands' and the 'unnecessary visits'. Even 'the ingratiating manner' can give rise to loathing and contempt in the heart of the genial family doctor. But, as soon as I recognise characters in the surgery as belonging to the same human family as my friends from the classics, my anger and frustration dissolve, and a nicer part of my personality is able to emerge. If you were to call all this an enhanced capacity for empathy, I should not disagree. But do I have any greater insight into my patients' souls? Does the wisdom and insight of the great writers help me to a better understanding of human emotions and behaviour? I hope so and I would certainly maintain that a writer like Tolstoy (when he is writing fiction) can tell you more about what it is to be human and have feelings than any number of textbooks of psychology or handbooks of psychotherapy.

More recently I began to feel the need to share my enjoyment of reading the classics with my colleagues. I requested, and was given (by an enlightened editor), the opportunity to write a regular column on medicine and literature in the quarterly journal *Education for Primary Care* (formerly *Education for General Practice*). In each issue, the column consists mainly of an in-depth account of one of my favourite classics. The aim is to invite people who have never read the book to give it a try and to encourage those who read it years ago and remember it vaguely to read it again. I also invite guest writers to contribute articles about their favourite books. These articles have now been collected and published, with some revisions and additions, in the present book.

Do doctors have time to read books for pleasure? When I ask my colleagues and GP registrars I am pleased to find that most of them are quietly reading all sorts of non-medical books. Mostly they read recently published books, and my friends sometimes ask me why I chose only to write about the classics. The answer is that they are so much better written than most other books. Clearly they have shown their quality simply by surviving while numerous others, published at the same time, have vanished without trace. The high quality of the classics is evident in their sheer reliability. If you are going on a long plane journey, choosing a book from the airport book shop is risky: you may end up tossing it aside in irritation after a few pages. But a classic will not let you down. Pack something like *War and Peace* in your flight bag and, although you may have to work at it a bit to get into the story, you will soon be happily absorbed and oblivious to discomfort, delays and appalling food.

Italo Calvino the Italian writer (whose brilliant novel *If on a Winter's Night, a Traveller* is included in my selection) wrote an essay called 'Why Read the Classics?' Calvino offers 14 reasons for reading the classics, of which I find number nine the most interesting: 'Classics are books which, the more we know them through hearsay, the more original, unexpected, and innovative we find them when we actually read them.' He goes on to say that there has to be 'a spark' between reader and book; there is no point in reading the classics out of a sense of duty or respect, we should only read them for love. The exception is reading at school; school has to teach you to know (whether you like it or not) a number of classics, some of which you will later recognise as 'your classics'.

The books discussed here are, of course, those which are special for me and for my guests. It may surprise you to find that most of them are not about medical subjects. When I mention my interest in the classics to professors of literature, they are, of course, pleased to hear about it, but they tend to assume that I am only concerned with stories about doctors. I have to assure them that this is not the case. It is true that we can learn a great deal from stories about doctors, if only about how badly they can behave. Fictional accounts of doctors and their patients can provide excellent teaching material for students and I shall say something about the place of literature in the medical school a little further on. But I wanted to feel free to include my favourite classics regardless of whether they had doctors as principal characters.

Of course, even when they are not the main focus of attention, doctors have a way of creeping in at the margins of literature: it is difficult to keep them out. When they do appear, I find them fascinating, as I guess all doctors do, and I am happy to spend some time with them. They are colleagues after all: we want to compare our practices with theirs and cheer them on when they do something decent or noble. Unfortunately, most literary doctors show a dismaying lack of moral fibre, decency or even professional competence. The only truly heroic fictional doctors seem to be those who appear in novels written by doctors themselves.

But if you are looking for ordinary, frail, human doctors you will find plenty of them popping up to diagnose and prognosticate in the books we talk about here: there is Emily Brontë's Dr Kenneth, who does his best with some very difficult patients in *Wuthering Heights*; we have Dr Slop the man-midwife, who makes a botched delivery of the infant Tristram Shandy (breaking his poor little nose in the process); and, talking of obstetrics, we spend an evening in the Dublin Rotunda Hospital in the company of Leopold Bloom and a crowd of drunken medical students. We study the career of young Dr Lydgate (of *Middlemarch*) in some detail and emerge shaking our heads sadly. And of course, the collection begins with Kafka's unnamed Country Doctor, who is whirled away by magical horses on the 'Night Call from Hell'.

As you scan the contents page, you may be wondering how and why these particular works were chosen. You will observe that they are arranged in no particular order, either chronological or thematic. They were chosen because they are favourites with a special meaning for me or for my guests, and because they are classics. They present themselves, more or less, in the order in which they appeared in the Medicine and Literature column. I began with Kafka's short story *A Country Doctor* because of a quotation from it which has acquired a special significance for GPs: 'To write prescriptions is easy, but coming to an understanding with people is hard.' And also because I thought that a story about a GP would entice a few of my colleagues who 'have no time for reading' to give it a try (it is only six pages long). The next piece, on *A Midsummer Night's Dream*, was inspired by the need to explain to my group of GP registrars why their course organiser was taking them to see a Shakespeare play. After that came some of the big books which sit beside my bed, ready for me to reread a chapter or two (at random) whenever I feel the need to revisit my friends within. They include *Anna Karenin, Mansfield Park, Wuthering Heights* and *Tess of the d'Urbervilles.* Some of my choices have a reputation for being difficult or obscure. James Joyce's *Ulysses*, perhaps the greatest twentieth-century novel in English, seems to put off nearly everyone. So why do I love it so much? I try to explain why and hope that more readers will be encouraged to share in the fun. Another secret delight waiting to be discovered is Laurence Sterne's *Tristram Shandy.* Anything written in the eighteenth century may seem very remote to a modern reader, but not this book, which is amazingly modern (or even post-modern) and full of wonderful comic scenes, delightful characters and, of course, digressions.

Not all the books were chosen by me: it is a pleasure to welcome some of my friends and fellow classics readers who have contributed to the column and now the book. Brian Glasser has written about Hemingway's story *Indian Camp*, which graphically exposes the non-empathetic doctor and ends so tragically. Oliver Samuel leads us very happily into an appreciation of the sonnets of Shakespeare and Donne; Tim Swanwick celebrates the life and work of Mikhail Bulgakov, a country doctor who also happened to be a literary genius; and Gillie Bolton treats us to an exploration of *The Rime of the Ancient Mariner.*

All the chapters have been written chiefly with the aim of sharing and spreading the pleasure of reading the classics to our fellow doctors, who work terribly hard and are in desperate need of a little spiritual refreshment. And if one of these books becomes one of 'your classics' it will stay with you for life as a constant inner resource whenever you begin to despair of the human race. Will 'your classics' help you to be a better doctor? I make no promises and you may already be a better doctor. I don't insist on the classics earning their living in this way. They are simply there, like the mountains and the stars, to give lasting pleasure to everyone who discovers them.

All the same, if the classics can have a beneficial effect on the professional persona, we should surely be introducing them to students as part of the curriculum. Unhappily, most medical students are still deprived of literature from an early age, as soon as they are segregated into the scientific side of the educational system. But this situation can be remedied. There is now a growing interest in many medical schools in the teaching of the humanities as applied to medicine. Literature, and especially classic literature, has an important part to play in this new curriculum and it is my hope that this book will prove helpful to those of my colleagues who are enthusiastically bringing reading back into medical studies. GP registrars might also benefit from the introduction of some literature into the half-day release course; some courses already include 'book review' sessions and I have tried them myself with some encouraging results. In the final chapter of this book, I discuss some of the ways in which the books described here might be used for teaching purposes.

I would like to thank my guest writers for their valuable contribution of voices different from mine; I am also grateful to Alistair Stead for his expert guidance and constructive suggestions. He has also provided three valuable contributions in the form of 'postscripts', which shed a different light on the books and gently counterbalance some of my errors and omissions.

I would like to thank the editors of *Education for Primary Care*, Declan Dwyer and John Pitts, for their encouragement with the original 'Medicine and Literature' section of the journal in which these articles first appeared; and everyone who has written to me and told me that they have enjoyed one of my classics as a result of reading an account of it in the journal. It is my hope that all of you will find yourselves heading for the library or the bookshop or perhaps just dusting off a few neglected volumes from your own shelves. I want to see you all, in my imagination, settling down happily with a copy of a classic book and, for a couple of hours, forgetting all the tedious vexations which beset the National Health Service. I feel confident that you will emerge refreshed and invigorated and with smiles on your faces. But what should you read first? In the following pages my friends and I will be happy to offer some suggestions.

Reference

Calvino I (1991) *Why Read the Classics?* Translation by Martin McLaughlin (1999). Vintage, Random House, London.

2

A Country Doctor

a short story by Franz Kafka

I first came across a reference to Franz Kafka's story *A Country Doctor*[1] about 25 years ago, when I was starting out in general practice and thus becoming a 'country doctor' myself. I can't remember the exact context, but I know that it was quoted in an article by Marshall Marinker, one of the pioneers of the New British General Practice of the early 1970s. When I telephoned Marshall to ask him about it, he told me he had first used the quotation as an epigraph on the title page of a book called *Treatment or Diagnosis*,[2] of which he was a co-author. The book is an account of a study of the 'repeat prescription' patient by one of Michael Balint's research groups. And the quotation was: 'To write prescriptions is easy, but to come to an understanding with people is hard.'

Brilliant! I thought, and no doubt lots of other idealistic young GPs thought so too, for I kept hearing the phrase quoted at educational meetings. It was a wise saying from a famous writer, which encapsulated everything we stood for. Our mission as family doctors was (and is) not just to scribble on the pad but to connect with our patients as human beings, experience the spark of empathy and mobilise our resources, both human and medical – and to reach out to them with compassion, insight and wisdom.

A couple of years later, I was wandering around Oxford with Philip Hopkins, who is another pioneer GP and founder of the Balint Society. In the window of a second-hand bookshop,

we came across a beautiful edition, illustrated with woodcuts, of
A Country Doctor by Franz Kafka. 'Look there,' I said to Philip,
'that's the story with the famous quotation about writing pre-
scriptions being easy. It's one of general practice's special books.'
We went inside, examined the book and enquired about the price.
I remember that it was in German and that it was very expensive.
I decided (foolishly) that I didn't want it that much. But Philip
bought it. I wonder if he still has it.

When I got home I bought a Penguin edition of Kafka's stories
and actually read *A Country Doctor* myself for the first time. I was
knocked out by its power and its vivid dream-like strangeness. I
suppose I had been expecting some sort of Czech–Jewish version
of *Dr Finlay's Casebook*, with a wise old doctor giving an eager
youngster the benefit of his experience. I should have known
better. I had, after all, read *The Trial* and *Metamorphosis*: I knew that
Kafka wasn't like that. So what happens in this famous story?
And what does it mean? Does it truly have a take-home message
for real-life country doctors like us?

Here's how it goes. The doctor has received an urgent night call
to a patient in a village ten miles away. It is snowing a blizzard
and the doctor's horse has died in the night so he has no means
of transport. Striding around his courtyard in 'confused distress',
he kicks at the door of a disused pigsty. The door flies open to
reveal two magnificent horses and a strange groom, who offers to
yoke them up and get his gig ready. Unfortunately, this groom
also has evil designs on the doctor's servant girl, Rose. Before
he knows what is happening, the doctor finds that the horses
are carrying him away in the gig and the last thing he sees is the
groom battering down the door of his house in order to get at
the terrified Rose, who has locked herself inside. The reader is
now, like the doctor, overwhelmed with dismay, carried off by the
galloping horses and gazing back in horror. The night call has
become a nightmare; how can a doctor concentrate on his patient
when frightful things are happening at home which are totally
out of his control?

Surprisingly, the journey takes no time at all; the doctor's
courtyard seems to open directly into the patient's farmyard. The
horses are still, the snow has stopped and the scene is bathed in

moonlight (this is a very visual story; it would make a wonderful film. I see Gene Hackman as the doctor and Jack Nicholson as the groom. As for Rose: Kate Winslett? Nicole Kidman? You choose). Now the patient's parents are hurrying the doctor into the house; their son is a gaunt young man without a shirt, who throws his arms round the doctor's neck and says, 'Let me die'. The doctor opens his bag and fiddles about with his instruments while the relatives watch and wait (the way they do). Even the two horses are watching him, each with its head poked through a window – another wonderful image. The doctor is preoccupied with his own problems. The family observe his discomfort and try to make him feel at ease: the sister takes his fur coat and the father offers him a glass of rum, which he refuses. (We all know this scene, don't we? We've been in bedrooms like this with the relatives crowding around expectantly, trying to help, driving you crazy.) But how does Kafka know? Had he ever been on a night call, or is this sheer imagination? One clue I found in a biography of Kafka,[3] is that Kafka had an Uncle Siegfried, a slim, slightly crazy, bird-like man *who was a country doctor*! As a young man, Kafka sometimes stayed with him and enjoyed peaceful country holidays, but did he ever accompany his uncle on his visits?

Now the doctor lays his wet, bearded face on the boy's chest (couldn't find his stethoscope, apparently) and decides that he is healthy, nothing the matter with him. Another totally inappropriate night call, he thinks. And he goes on ruminating angrily about how unreasonable and ungrateful patients are. They know nothing about his own horrible situation and if they did, they wouldn't believe it. This is where the famous quotation comes: 'Writing prescriptions is easy, but coming to an understanding with people is hard.' In context, it seems as though he is pleading for the patients to understand him, in a rather self-pitying way. The fact that they torment him with their ringing of his night bell is bad enough, but now he is going to have to sacrifice Rose as well. Just what is his relationship with Rose? You want to know, and so do I. She is the 'lovely girl who'd lived in my house for years without my hardly noticing her'. That's all we're told about Rose; I find that word 'hardly' very poignant, aching with love that might have been. At one point our poor country doctor says that if the boy wants to die, then once he has sorted Rose out, he will be ready to die as well. He is clearly suffering from a serious degree of professional burnout amounting to clinical depression. He needs the services of a counselling helpline and, above all, to join the nearest out of hours co-operative so that the terrible burden of night calls can be lifted from his shoulders.

But is Kafka really writing about the problems endemic in a badly organised primary care service – or something else? We shall return to those considerations later on, but now, the crucial (and I mean crucial) part of the story is approaching. The doctor is about to go when he realises that the family will be devastated if he leaves them after such a cursory examination. The mother is tearful and the sister is fluttering a blood-soaked towel or hand-kerchief. Wisely, he decides to examine the patient properly and this time he discovers THE WOUND. Yes, in the boy's right side there is a ghastly wound 'as big as the palm of my hand'. The wound is 'rose-red' in colour (reminding us of the doctor's wounded 'Rose' back home). And it is crawling with worms, which, and I hate to have to tell you this, have little legs. Maybe Kafka is piling on the horror a bit too much there, but legs or no legs, the description is enough to chill the stomach. Instantly, the doctor realises that the young man is incurable, doomed. We doctors all know that moment, don't we? We have recognised the presence of Death in a patient's physical signs but we have yet to speak. Now the doctor realises that the patient was right after all. This sort of thing has happened to me and I dare say to you too. Why do we make these mistakes? Are we too afraid of the awful truth of mortality to confront it until the patient insists that we look again?

In any event, the family are now pleased with the doctor and the boy whispers, 'Will you save me?' Our unhappy GP feels ex-asperated because they expect him to cure the boy. 'They expect the impossible,' he grumbles. But strange things begin to happen. The family and the village elders all seize the doctor and strip off his clothes. (This has, in all probability, not happened to any of us in the course of a night call. Or perhaps it has metaphorically.) A village children's choir appears outside the house (another nice cinematic touch) and start to sing ('Strip him naked, then he'll heal us; should he fail to, kill him quick!'). The naked doctor finds himself thrust into bed with his patient. Everyone goes away (except the two horses) and silence falls. Doctor and patient, side by side in bed, begin a strange dialogue. At first the boy is bitter and petulant: 'I don't have much confidence in you. Instead of helping, you're cramping my deathbed. I'd like best to scratch your eyes out.' The doctor agrees that he has been quite inadequate and asks for some consideration ('… it's none too easy for me either.') The boy becomes resigned to his fate: 'I came into the world with a fine wound; that's all I have to my name.' Now, in a disturbing change of tack, the doctor starts to use false reassurance. He boasts about his wide clinical experience and declares that, actually, the boy's wound is not too bad. The sort of thing that could easily be acquired from an accident with an axe in the forest. Is he telling the patient he is going to live after all? It is not quite clear, but it is certainly a piece of bare-faced hypocrisy and denial. Doctors used to lie to dying patients all the time, but we are now taught to be more honest if we can. And that means being brave, because we have to die one day as well, in spite of having gone into medicine to avoid it.

Anyway, the patient is reassured for the moment, and the doctor seizes his chance to escape. He hurriedly gathers up his clothes, his bag and his fur coat and throws them into the gig (presumably through the window) as one of the horses backs away. The fur coat misses but catches on a hook at the back of the gig by one sleeve. The fleeing doctor jumps on to one of the horses and tries to drive the whole outfit home as fast as he can. But this time there is no galloping; the horses move with agonising deliberation as if in slow motion. As they crawl interminably through the snowy wastes, the doctor continues to wail about his fate: he'll never get home, his practice is done for, the disgusting groom is raping poor Rose, he is old, naked and helpless; he can't even reach his fur coat which is trailing along in the snow. The final sentence: 'Respond to a false alarm on the night bell – and it can't be made good, ever again.'

I find that despairing ending puzzling. I find the whole story puzzling as well as disturbing and exhilarating. Can the decision to go on a night visit really change your life irrevocably for the worse? I can think of a few that have influenced me profoundly and made me question what I was about; but none that has led to such an irreversible fall from grace. And why does the doctor call it 'a false alarm' when he agrees in the end that the patient is mortally ill? It would be nice to be able to ask our poor colleague a few questions. Yes, he really seems to be a colleague by the time we've finished his story. And yet, although this story has a great fascination for real-life country doctors, I can't help feeling that Kafka didn't really write it just for our benefit. He must have had other fish to fry, which for him were more important (if you can get your mind round the concept of anything being more important than a doctor's problems).

I decided that, in order to deepen my understanding of *A Country Doctor* (which had begun to exert a obsessive hold on my attention), I needed to consult a literary expert. I telephoned my friend Alistair Stead, who teaches English literature at the University of Leeds. Yes, he knew the story, it was one of Kafka's best. After a pause, in which he re-read the story (it is only about six pages), he called me back and told me a lot more about it, none of which had much to do with doctors. I will try and convey something of what he told me but I may get some of it wrong and miss out something really important. You (and he) will have to forgive me. The first thing to understand is that the story has to be read on many different levels; it is a straightforward narrative (more or less) and it is also a fantastic dream full of non-sequiturs and surreal juxtapositions. It is full of symbols, which invite psycho-analytic or even theological interpretations.

Kafka saw himself as an artist under a compulsion (inner or outer) to express himself in writing and to do justice to his gifts. He hated theories and wanted to communicate profoundly serious thoughts and feelings without preaching to his readers or moralising ('Writing prescriptions is easy …'). Throughout his life he felt himself to be crushed by his dominating father who had little respect for his son's writing talent. ('Just put it on my bedside table,' he said when the young Franz proudly showed him an advance copy of *A Country Doctor*.) In the story, the anguished young patient with his fatal wound ('a fine wound; that's all I have to my name') reminds us of Franz agonising over his painful, perhaps fatal, literary responsibility. The doctor, the older man, comfortably off with his fur coat, suggests Kafka's father. But, ironically, the two are pressed up against one another in the bed and the father/doctor takes on some of his literary son's attributes: he is a healing artist, uncomfortably aware of the need to rise to the world's and his own expectations. On yet another level, that terrible wound in the side reminds us of Jesus Christ being crucified; or is it Kafka who is being crucified? Does he see himself as a Christ figure, redeeming the world through his art? At each 'level' of interpretation there is a tension between a youth and an older man: Kafka and his father, the old doctor and the young patient, and the crucified Jesus and His Father. The story is so brilliantly constructed that all these levels, the medical, the familial, the artistic and the religious, come together in appearing to allude to someone who assumes an awesome responsibility (Alistair's phrase) to care for or cure the world. It is also impossible to forget (once you know it) that Kafka died prematurely from incurable tuberculosis. It is true that he didn't have his first haemoptysis (which told him that he would never reach old age or even maturity) until a year after he wrote *A Country Doctor*, but he may have had a premonition: tuberculosis was common.

In the course of our phone conversation, Alistair and I also talked about Kafka and sexuality. He never managed to get himself married, although it was something he greatly wished for. He was engaged to Felice Bauer twice and had another important relationship (with Milena Jesenská) later on. Only when he was close to dying did he achieve a brief fulfilment with Dora Dymant. The greater part of his relationship with both Felice and Milena was carried out through letters. Sexuality both fascinated and repelled him: I think he found it very scary, although he was very attracted to women. (Poor little Rose must be in there somewhere.) Those wonderful animals, the two horses, must symbolise the power of sexuality, and the lascivious groom suggests some sort of horror and fear aroused by sexual desires out of control. Alistair and I also talked about the ending of the story and whether it is totally despairing. He thought there were some hopeful signs that the doctor does not see himself as having failed completely. But you must read it for yourself and see what you think.

The more I read *A Country Doctor* the more things I find in it to treasure and to wonder at. It is very short, little more than a fragment, but not a word is wasted. At the end of my investigation I still don't really understand what it means, but that no longer matters because I feel that there is a lot in it that I can understand. I do think it has 'take-home messages' for us country doctors. It works as a story about a real doctor, although it's even better if you are aware of some of the figurative threads running through it as well. Somehow, Kafka, while going about all his other important business in the story, manages to get to the heart of how we doctors feel when people cry to us for help and tug at our clothes, look reproachfully at us and always (it seems) at the wrong time, when we have important personal stuff to attend to. We recognise the exasperation, the guilt, the feeling of responsibility leading to the decision to try again, to lower the defences, to share the pain. There is even, in the way the story is told, a sense of the love that country doctors have for those pesky peasant-patients.

I feel a little sad that we family doctors are now rapidly shedding as much out-of-hours work as we can so that the horrible house call in the middle of the night and the emotions it arouses may become part of history. Future editions of *A Country Doctor* may need to include a footnote to explain that country doctors used to do house calls.

The text

A Country Doctor by Franz Kafka was probably written in 1916 and published as the title story of a collection of short stories in the autumn of 1919. Kafka died of tuberculosis in 1924 at the age of 41.

The quotations used in this chapter are from the translation by Iain Bamforth (himself a country doctor), which was published in the *British Journal of General Practice* (1999), **50**: 1036–1039. They are reprinted by kind permission of Dr Bamforth.

References

1 *A Country Doctor* can also be found in Kafka F, *The Trans-formation ('Metamorphosis') and Other Stories*. Translation by Malcolm Pasley (1992). Penguin, Harmondsworth.

2 Balint M, Hunt N, Joyce D, Marinker M, Woodcock J (1970) *Treatment or Diagnosis; a study of repeat prescriptions in general practice*. Tavistock Publications, London.

3 Citati P (1990) *Kafka*. Translation by R Rosenthal. Martin, Secker & Warburg, London.

3

A Midsummer Night's Dream

by William Shakespeare

Prologue

One summer, I decided that it would be nice to take my group of GP registrars to a play as an end-of-term treat. To my secret satisfaction, out of the three options I gave them, they chose Shakespeare's *A Midsummer Night's Dream* at the Open Air Theatre in Regent's Park, London. I firmly believed, then as now, that a medical education should include a dose of the humanities if we are to be humane doctors; and no one understood humanity better than Shakespeare.

However, one or two of the GP registrars were unable to see how watching a play with no discernible medical content could be justified as part of the curriculum. And another, perhaps feeling apprehensive about being suddenly exposed to high literary culture, asked if I could explain it to them before we went. So I decided to devote part of the afternoon before we went to the theatre to an exposition of *The Dream*, which would include an account of the important messages I felt sure it must contain for GPs everywhere. I had seen the play myself a number of times and always enjoyed it, but my recollection of the plot was hazy. When I looked up the file in my brain it said: 'Funny play by Shakespeare. Always willing to see it but no more amateur or school productions please. Play concerns conflict between fairies and mortals. Fairies have gossamer dresses and dance around to Mendelssohn music. Mischievous goblin character called Puck teases mortals and makes them fall asleep. When they wake up they fall in love with the wrong people. Fairy Queen falls in love with comic yokel called Bottom to whom Puck has given a donkey's head. Then Bottom and the other peasants put on a play which is very comical. All ends happily.' You probably recognise the play now and have a similar file on it yourselves. My next task was to read the text, which I did – and I really enjoyed it for all sorts of reasons which I'll try to make clear to you. I can't really divide it into characters, plot, themes, images, etc. I'm not here to write an A-level guide, I hope. I think I'll just take you with me into the play until you don't need me any more and you become impatient to read it for yourselves. And, of course, to go and see it.

The Dream teams

The Dream has three entirely different teams of characters: there are the upper-class Athenians, the lower-class tradesmen (who are keen amateur actors) and, of course, the fairies. The first three scenes conveniently introduce each of the teams and set three interweaving plots in motion.

The opening scene

The play starts with Theseus, the Duke of Athens, having a conversation with his bride-to-be, Hippolyta, Queen of the Amazons. I don't suppose you remember these two, and just where they are coming from is a bit of a puzzle. We are supposed to be in Athens, but there are no reference points to ancient Greece and we might as well be in Athens, Georgia. And although these two are quite happily anticipating their forthcoming wedding, it appears from something that Theseus lets slip ('Hippolyta, I wooed thee with my sword') that he originally acquired her by military conquest, which gives me a slight feeling of discomfort. Best not to worry too much though, because she seems to be making the best of it and something else is happening to distract us. Enter a courtier, an elderly man called Egeus, who complains to the Duke that his daughter (Hermia) is in love with the wrong boy. He wants her to marry Demetrius but she prefers another young man called Lysander. He complains that Lysander has 'bewitched the bosom of my child' by singing at her window by moonlight and sending her 'bracelets of thy hair, rings, gauds, conceits, knacks, trifles, nosegays, sweetmeats'. Hermia herself appears and tells her father she would rather die a virgin than marry Demetrius. The two young men also appear and we are totally engrossed in the emotional conflicts of all the characters.

The Duke sides with the enraged father, and rules that if Hermia disobeys her old man she must either die or spend the rest of her life in a convent. Poor Hermia is on the verge of tears and Lysander observes that 'the course of true love never did run smooth'. One of the pleasures of reading Shakespeare is that you keep stumbling across well-known quotations in their original context and greeting them with little cries of pleasure (well, I do, anyway). There will be lots more, some of which I shall gleefully point out to you. Meanwhile, our young lovers have decided to run away and meet secretly in the forest. At this point Hermia's old school chum Helena appears. Now she is besotted with Demetrius (Hermia's rejected suitor, you remember), with whom she once had an understanding. She keeps pursuing Demetrius but he rather cruelly ignores her. Helena decides that she will let Demetrius know that Hermia is running off to the forest so that he will follow her – and she will follow him.

The scene ends. Our imagination is caught and held by a good dramatic story, told, I need hardly say, in wonderful Shakespearean verse. Would I had space to quote more – be assured that that there are more samples to come when we get to my most favourite bits.

The rude mechanicals

But now the next team have taken over the stage: the comic Athenian tradesmen who speak in prose to show that they are working class. They are evidently about to rehearse a play (within the play) called *Pyramus and Thisbe*, a comical tragedy about star-crossed lovers. (It is interesting that Shakespeare was writing *Romeo and Juliet* at about the same time as *The Dream*.) The director of this amateur dramatic society, Peter Quince, calls out his members' names and allocates their parts. They all have lovely names such as Flute the Bellows Mender, Snug the Joiner and Snout the Tinker. And, of course, Nick Bottom, the weaver, who reckons he knows at least as much about the theatre as Quince and keeps interrupting with helpful suggestions. It is a familiar situation to all course organisers and Quince handles it brilliantly. He is terribly patient even when Bottom wants to play all the parts. He values everyone's contribution but stays firmly in control of the group. Finally Bottom accepts the main part of Pyramus, the lover of Thisbe. They arrange to meet in the woods (yes, the same woods) by moonlight to start rehearsing. 'We will meet,' says Bottom solemnly, 'and there we will rehearse most obscenely and courageously. Take pains; be perfect.' So now Will Shakespeare has set up two teams of characters converging on the woods with different agendas. But there is another team we have almost forgotten about: it is time to meet, the fairies.

(We have reached Act 1 Scene 2 in the text. All Shakespeare's plays had five acts, probably to promote the sales of comfits and sweetmeats in the four intervals. When you go to see it there will just be one interval in the middle.)

Fairies

Enter a fairy at one door and Robin Goodfellow at the other. The fairy and her colleagues (who have names like Peaseblossom and Mustard Seed) may be in ballet frocks or, in modern productions, all kinds of strange gear. Robin Goodfellow, more often known as Puck, is a knowing sprite or hobgoblin. He is personal assistant to Oberon, King of the Fairies, who soon makes his appearance. He and his Queen, Titania, are in the middle of a spot of marital coolness when we met them. Both of them want possession of 'a little Indian boy' whom Titania has adopted and Oberon fancies as – well, we had better not go into why Oberon fancies him. Let's just say it is a child custody battle without the benefit of social workers. When the two encounter each other on the stage, Oberon cries: 'Ill met by moonlight, proud Titania.' Wouldn't you love to be able to say that to someone in the middle of a wood on a moonlit night? And she replies: 'What, jealous Oberon? – Fairies, skip hence. I have forsworn his bed and company.' Titania goes on to complain that their fairy quarrel has upset the rhythm of the seasons and caused various natural disasters. Oberon says all can be resolved if she will just give way. Typical of a man you might think. But Titania won't give way and she sweeps off with her retinue of fairies.

Now Oberon has a very important conversation with Puck. He tells his faithful assistant to fetch him a special flower called Love-in-Idleness (it is actually a Pansy), which has magic properties:

> *The juice of it on sleeping eyelids laid*
> *Will make or man or woman madly dote*
> *Upon the next live creature that it sees.*

And Puck races off to pluck the flower with the immortal words: 'I'll put a girdle round about the earth in forty minutes.' While he is gone, the first of the mortals appear in the woods and Oberon takes an interest in their affairs. He sees that Helena is in love with Demetrius, who is rejecting her. When Puck comes back with the eye drops (as we doctors call them), Oberon instructs him to give a dose to Demetrius (now conveniently asleep) so that he will fall in love with Helena as soon as he wakes up and sees her. Meanwhile, Oberon will administer the magic drops to Titania, his fairy Queen, so that she will fall in love with – who knows what? The idea is to humiliate her and teach her a lesson

> *With the juice of this I'll streak her eyes*
> *And fill her full of hateful fantasies.*

He is a bit of a bastard, really, that Oberon. But he has a way with words, and I must quote you the following:

> I know a bank where the wild thyme blows
> Where oxlips and the nodding violet grows,
> Quite overcanopied with luscious woodbine,
> With sweet musk-roses and with eglantine.
> There sleeps Titania sometime of the night
> Lulled in these flowers with dances and delight.

Isn't that gorgeous? I love the idea of Titania being 'sometime of the night'; it is a very sexy description.

The rest of the plot (in a cowslip's ear)

Now things get really, really complicated. I don't have enough space to give you all the details of the rest of the plot, so we will summarise and pick out a few delicious moments. What happens next? Well, first of all, things go badly wrong with the eyedrop business because Puck mistakes Lysander, Hermia's true love, for Demetrius, and Lysander wakes up to fall in love with Helena. Puck realises his mistake and gives Demetrius a dose as well and we end up with both boys madly in love with Helena, who thought nobody loved her at all. She thinks they must be teasing her, but poor Hermia is very upset, as you can imagine. It really is a mess. But, I can reassure you, it does eventually get sorted out because in these magic woods people are constantly lying down and falling asleep so that it is possible for Puck to give the right drops to the right patient and for Oberon to supply an antidote.

Meanwhile the actors have met in the woods to rehearse. Puck spots them and says to himself: 'What hempen homespuns have we swagg'ring here?' (You should try that one when you come across a group of colleagues engaged in some well-meaning but pointless activity. And add, to mystify them totally: 'so near the cradle of the fairy Queen'.) Of course, the actors can't see or hear him because they are mortals and he is a fairy. Puck leads Bottom away and returns him to the group with an ass's head instead of his own human one. The other players scatter in consternation when they find their friend going 'Ee-ore!', as he does on stage, to great effect, often with a waggle of his animatronic ears. And now comes the central defining moment of the play. Bottom wanders into Titania's bower. She awakes and as he is the first 'thing' she espies, she is immediately in love with him. She takes him to her bed and decorates his hairy face with flowers while the fairies wait upon his every whim. Bottom acquiesces very happily. Titania behaves like a little girl in love with her pony: it is all quite understandable.

But it doesn't last long. Oberon lifts the spell with a quick application of the antidote eye drops, Titania come to her senses and Bottom gets his normal head back. He wanders through the wood in a bemused state until he encounters his companions, who are delighted to see him restored to his old self. But he's not quite the same. When they ask him to explain where he has been, he does so in the following amusing and wondrous meditation:

> *I have had a most rare vision. I have had a dream past the wit of man to say what dream it was. Man is but an ass if he go about to expound this dream. Methought I was – and methought I had – but a man is a patched fool if he will offer to say what methought I had. The eye of man hath not heard, the ear of man hath not seen, man's hand is not able to taste, his tongue to conceive, nor his heart to report on what my dream was. I will get Peter Quince to write a ballad of this dream. It shall be called "Bottom's Dream" because it hath no bottom ...*

In the last act, the tradesmen perform their play for the entertainment of the Duke and his friends. It is usually hysterically funny with lots of inspired comic business, but obviously you have to see it to appreciate that. The young lovers are happily and appropriately paired off and all is forgiven. Or is it? Puck addresses the audience at the end and asks the audience's pardon for all the tricks that have been played on them:

> *If we shadows have offended*
> *Think but this, and all is mended:*
> *That you have but slumbered here*
> *While these visions did appear.*

Was it all a dream then? It can certainly seem like one if you see a good production and especially in the magical outdoor setting of the Regents Park Open Air Theatre on a summer evening. But what are the educational take-home messages for the busy GP?

The play's messages for the busy GP

1   It deals with a number of *human relationship problems*, which frequently trouble our patients. These include child custody conflicts, the heavy father who objects to his daughter's chosen lover, love unrequited and feelings subjected to ridicule.

2   *Team building.* Peter Quince demonstrates facilitating skills in getting his team of amateur actors to work together, despite their conflicting demands and personalities.

3   *Exercise great care* in the use of eye drops! Shakespeare shows how it is all too easy for the inexperienced practitioner to produce unwanted effects by the injudicious use of powerful eye medication.

4   *Bottom's dream: the therapeutic magic of the doctor–patient relationship.* There are occasions when patients feel better just because the doctor has listened carefully, given them some precious professional attention and made them feel that she cares. They come away from such a consultation feeling better without really knowing why. I think that something of this sort happens to Bottom when, in a brief dream consultation, he has the experience of being loved and cared for by Titania.

Brush up your Shakespeare

So take your registrars (or your students) to see *A Midsummer Night's Dream*. It is bound to be on somewhere this summer. If not, any Shakespeare play will do. I can think of no better way to top up a medical education.

The text

I used the Oxford World's Classic edition of *A Midsummer Night's Dream;* The New Penguin Shakespeare series is also very good but many people say that the Arden Shakespeare provides the most comprehensive introduction and notes.

4

Anna Karenin

by Lev Tolstoy

Count Lev Tolstoy is probably the greatest of the nineteenth-century Russian novelists. He was born in 1828 and died in 1910 at a railway station, trying to run away from home at the age of 82. During the course of a long and tempestuous life he was a soldier, a country landowner, a farmer and a teacher; a man with overwhelming sexual appetites who also suffered terrible guilt feelings; the father of a large family and an impossible husband whose wife stuck with him faithfully to the end; a visionary and religious zealot who tried desperately to lead a Christ-like existence. Most important of all (although he wouldn't have thought so) he was an incredibly gifted writer who could bring his characters to such vibrant life that you feel you know them personally. As far as I know, he never studied medicine like his younger contemporary Dr Chekhov; and yet *Anna Karenin* could serve admirably as a textbook of medical humanities for family doctors. It contains descriptions of all the important events in life which we are called upon to witness: falling in love, love unrequited, psychosomatic illness, parental anxiety about adolescent children, marriage, childbirth, death in the family, adultery and family break-up, jealousy, nervous breakdown, suicide and struggling to discover the meaning and purpose of it all.

The article that follows will, I hope, connect or reconnect you to *Anna Karenin*. I've also asked my friend Alistair Stead, who knows much more about Tolstoy and literature than I ever will (he can read it in Russian, for God's sake), to add a few words at the end so that we can also see it from the perspective of a professional. Alistair and I first met when we were students together nearly 30 years ago. He is now senior lecturer in English literature at the University of Leeds, whereas I, as you know, am just a humble country doctor. But we have stayed friends. When you have finished reading what he and I have to say, go into your study, or wherever you keep your books, and get down that old copy of *Anna Karenin*. Blow the dust off and settle down with it in your favourite armchair. I shall see that you are not disturbed ...

This is one of my most treasured books. It sits by my bedside so that any time I feel like it, I can pick it up and read a few chapters. Sometimes I just open it anywhere at random – I know it well enough to pick up the story at any point. Other nights I might re-read one of the special chapters to which I have awarded a rosette (more about them later). Why is this book so special for me and, I'm sure, lots of other people? Let's just refresh everyone's memory about it.

Anna Karenin (or *Karenina* if you prefer) was written in the 1870s by Russian author Lev Tolstoy, who also wrote *War and Peace*. You may have read it in your teens, as I did, and not been very impressed. Or at least it made an impression but was then put away somewhere on a seldom-visited mental bookshelf, just one of a large number of classics, mostly heavy and Russian, which our elders and tutors said we ought to have read. It is possible that you haven't read it at all (you can be honest), but you may have some idea of the story from seeing one of the several failed movie versions (the one with Greta Garbo is worth seeing). You will remember that Anna K is a beautiful, passionate, married woman who has a tempestuous affair with a young officer called Vronsky. Her husband refuses a divorce, the couple are ostracised by polite society and Anna finally commits suicide under the wheels of a train. You may also remember that there is another story, running alongside the Anna–Vronsky tragedy and interweaving with it. This concerns a young landowner called Levin, who falls in love with and eventually marries a sweet young thing called Kitty. Levin and Kitty have a much quieter life in the country and apart from the usual quarrels that young couples have, they seem to be very happy, despite Levin's tendency to brood about the Meaning of Life.

That's probably as much as you remember, isn't it? So let's look at the book afresh and I'll try to show you why I think it is quite wonderful and has the ability to make me feel good inside just from reading one or two chapters at random. I don't read Russian, regretfully, so we are going to use one of the English translations. The one I like best is the Penguin translation by Rosemary Edmonds. The book is divided into eight parts (I think it was originally published in instalments) and each part has 30 or so chapters, except for the last, which is much shorter. The chapters are all quite short, which is one reason I can easily read one or two before I go to sleep. Let's open the book at Part 1, Chapter 1, and see what we find. First of all, the famous opening sentence: 'All happy families are alike but an unhappy family is unhappy after its own fashion.' Is it true? Does it matter? Let's leave that for now and go on to the next two sentences: 'Everything had gone wrong in the Oblonsky household. The wife had found out about her husband's relationship with their former French governess.' Now Tolstoy has really grabbed our attention. A husband, a wife and a French governess – we want to know more.

Reading on, we are introduced to Prince Stepan Oblonsky (known to his friends as Stiva, or perhaps Steve would be better English). He is an easy-going, rather unserious, rather unfaithful but quite likeable member of the upper classes. A bit like Bertie Wooster but without Bertie's terror of sexuality. When we meet him, Stiva has just woken up from a pleasant dream and he stretches out his arm for his dressing gown, which should be hanging in its usual place beside his bed. But it's not there. Then he remembers with dismay that he has been sleeping not in the marital bed with his long-suffering wife Dolly, but on a morocco-leather couch in his study. Stiva is in the dog-house, in disgrace, because of that business with the French governess.

'"Oh dear, oh dear, oh dear," he groaned, remembering what had happened … "No she will never forgive me – she cannot forgive me and the worst of it is I am to blame for everything. I am to blame – and yet I am not to blame. That is the whole tragedy."' And he begins to review, unhappily, the events which have led him to this rude awakening on the morocco-leather couch. I have quoted all this in some detail because it illustrates the skill with which Tolstoy rapidly sketches in a character who then springs into life and engages our sympathy. And intense curiosity about what will happen next. Will she forgive him or not? And what has this to do with Anna Karenin? Have patience! Let's read on. Stiva gets up and tells us more about himself and Dolly. They have had seven children of whom five are still living. His wife is an excellent mother, but her good looks have faded and he is rather susceptible to younger women. His only regret is that he has been found out, because things had been going so well until that happened: she was happy with the children, and he could do what he liked.

He seeks counsel from his valet (I told you he was like Bertie Wooster), who tells him blandly that 'things will right themselves'. Then the children's nurse comes in and urges him to confess to Dolly that he is in the wrong. And if that doesn't work he should pray to the Lord. The one hopeful piece of news is that Stiva's sister Anna is coming for a visit. She will be able to save the marriage if anyone can. Yes, this is the famous Anna Karenin! She has yet to enter the story properly. She will arrive in Moscow by train in Chapter 18, when a chance meeting with Vronsky at the station will light the fuse of their affair. This awesome, heart-rending story lies ahead of us; but already we have been invited to meet Anna informally. She will come to her brother's house where, by now, we feel part of the family. We have sympathised with both Stiva and the offended Dolly; we have played with the children and we are hoping for everyone's sake that there will be a reconciliation. How does Tolstoy do it? How has he got us involved so quickly and effortlessly? Vladimir Nabokov in his *Lectures on Russian Literature* reckons that Tolstoy has a unique sense of time in his narrative style. 'He is the only writer I know of whose watch keeps time with the numberless watches of his readers.' However he does it, it works like a dream: as you read, the glass wall dissolves and you are just in there, along with the characters.

So what happens next? Well obviously I can't go through the whole book with you like this, but we'll do a bit more because it's fun, isn't it? Steve tries nervously to open negotiations with his wife but she cries bitterly and runs out, slamming the door behind her. The children are crying and everything is in chaos. It doesn't look good. Steve escapes to his office (he has a nice little government job which he actually does very competently) and afterwards meets his old friend Constantine, generally known by his surname Levin. Young Levin owns 6000 acres of farmland and lots of peasants, but he is a modest, unassuming chap who thinks a lot about life and just wants to do the right thing. Unlike his friend Steve, he's totally serious. I know you will like him.

Levin really hates the big city but has come up to town because he is seriously in love with a pretty blonde 18-year-old called Ekaterina Shcherbatsky. Her name is always shortened and anglicised by translators to Kitty. Which I think is absurd. Nobody is called Kitty these days, unless they are a cat. Her father calls her Katya or Katenka and it's obvious that we should call her Kate or Katie. I hope future translators will take note. Anyway, Katie or Kitty is, would you believe it, Dolly's little sister! So all these people are related and we begin to see why the story has begun with Steve who has a kind of pivotal position, linking by family ties the tragic Anna–Vronsky story and the more hopeful Levin–Kitty saga.

Levin has come up to Moscow expressly to propose to Kitty and he's very nervous. He thinks of her as 'mysterious, enchanting'. Actually she's just an ordinary kid like him and she's quite fond of him. We are coming up to the great skating scene (Chapter 9, one of the rosette winners). Levin has arrived at the Zoological Gardens, expecting to find Kitty there, because that's definitely the place to hang out if you want to skate and to be seen. He spots her family carriage at the gate and his heart starts thumping. Although the rink is full of skaters he recognises her at once: she's as easy to see 'as a rose among nettles'. And we are there too, sharing his joy and his terror, our hearts beating with his as we wait to see if she is going to be pleased to see him. She is! They skate together and she is impressed with his technique. He gets an invitation from her mother to come round to the house (or is it a palace?) on Thursday.

But the course of true love is always bumpy. It turns out that Kitty has also been receiving a good deal of attention from a young officer called Vronsky. Yes, the very same officer who will lead Anna to ecstasy and self-destruction. Of course Vronsky, with his arrogant good looks and his uniform, will be more attractive; even Kitty's mother, the Princess Shcherbatsky, is sufficiently carried away to hope for a marriage to him, although her father sees Vronsky for what he is and prefers Levin. So Levin psyches himself up to propose and Kitty turns him down with the words 'That cannot be'.

Poor Levin. We readers positively ache with sympathy for him. We have all been there, haven't we? Well, I know I have. Given the thumbs down by a fair-haired teenager who has got stars in her eyes about some football player. It's stupid, but it hurts. Never mind. It comes right in the end, for them at any rate. Kitty herself is eclipsed by Anna (who has dark curly hair falling over her beautiful white shoulders) at the famous ball scene (Chapter 22, rosette). Vronsky has eyes only for Anna and Kitty succumbs to a prolonged psychosomatic illness which worries her poor old Mum and Dad dreadfully. I need hardly tell you that the doctors are pompous and insensitive. Only the GP has a slight insight into the true nature of the illness (I'm straying ahead to Part 2 now). Levin meanwhile retires to his estate to commune with nature and learn some native wisdom from the peasants. Don't miss the amazing, sensuous description of Levin's day spent mowing with the farm workers. By the time you've read it your muscles will be aching, you'll feel the hot sun on your back and you'll need a long cool drink, but you'll have a wonderful contented glow (Part 3, Chapters 4 and 5, rosettes to both).

And so, after much heart searching on both sides, our young-sters meet again in Moscow the following year and this time everything goes right. Levin and Kitty communicate by chalking letters on a table and understand each other perfectly. They get married. They experience difficulties and disagreements but they overcome them. They cope with the death of Levin's difficult brother. They have a baby. Their life together is the story of any successful marriage but somehow all the more delightful for its ordinariness. Especially when it is contrasted every few chapters with the lives of Vronsky and Anna.

Before we meet Anna, Tolstoy gives us a little sketch of Vronsky. The first thing he tells us (Part 1, Chapter 16) is that 'Vronsky never really had a home-life.' His mother was a society woman, who had lots of affairs and clearly hadn't much time for her little boy, so it's not surprising that Vronsky is fairly cynical about love. He enjoys flirting with Kitty but has no intention of marrying her or anybody else. He is having too much fun with his regimental pals: going to parties, playing cards, getting a bit drunk.

In the next chapter, he goes, dutifully, to meet his old mother who is arriving by train from St Petersburg. At the station he sees Steve Oblonsky who is meeting his sister Anna on the same train. The two men watch as the steam locomotive comes in, making the platform vibrate with its power. The description is so good that we feel as if we too are waiting on the Moscow station platform on that fateful frosty morning. Then, as Vronsky is about to get in to his mother's compartment, he has to make way for a young woman getting out. He excuses himself and then does a double take because of the look she gives him with her 'brilliant grey eyes, shadowed with black lashes'. It is 'a friendly attentive look, as though she was recognising him'. The young woman is, of course, Anna, and it turns out that she and old Countess Vronsky have been sharing a compartment and having a long cosy chat. 'We have been talking about our sons, the whole time, I of mine and the Countess of hers', says Anna to Vronsky, 'and again a smile illumined her face, a caressing smile intended for him'.

Anna is a really lovely person. When she eventually arrives at Stiva and Dolly's she radiates a sort of sexy warmth and happiness so powerful that Dolly agrees to overlook her husband's misdemeanours one more time. And the children adore her. She and Vronsky meet again at the ball and dance together, but we only see them from a distance through the eyes of the wounded and jealous Kitty. A few days later, Anna is back at the station, saying to herself 'Well, that's all over, and thank heaven!'. She is on her way back to St Petersburg and is looking forward to being reunited with her little boy. But, in the train, she finds herself thinking about Vronsky again; she dozes off and has strange, frightening dreams. She wakes up to find the train has stopped at a station and there is a fierce snowstorm blowing. Anna gets out for a breath of fresh air and finds Vronsky on the platform. He has followed her on to the train back to Petersburg: 'I have to be where you are', he says, 'I can't help myself'. Something about Anna has hit Vronsky where it matters; he is no longer the rich little boy with no heart. And although Anna can be so wise and sensible and this is all madness, she has fallen just as deeply for him and there is no going back.

But life with Vronsky does not go smoothly. For a start her husband, the starchy civil servant Alexei Karenin, is not going to give her an inch. If she insists on running off with Vronsky he will not give her a divorce and (cruelly) will not let her have custody of their little son Seriozha. So poor Anna is forced to choose between lover and child. She chooses Vronsky, although her heart bleeds for her little boy. And we are forced to witness the effects on him of having his mother officially declared a non-person by his stern, angry father. Anna and Vronsky set up house together and defy society, which gives them a cold, unfeeling stare and looks away. It shouldn't matter, but it does. What matters even more is that Vronsky appears to be growing cold as well (or so it seems to Anna – we can never be sure). At any rate she becomes deeply unhappy and one day we realise with horror that she is comforting herself with opium. We witness her last, terrible days, culminating inevitably in her suicide at the same train station where she first met Vronsky.

And now we are going to have to stop. I realise I've been completely carried away by Anna and Levin and Kitty and the others and our time together is nearly up. I'm afraid I haven't been able to take you through the whole story in detail; but I hope I've been able to give you a few impressions of what it is like to enter Tolstoy's world and live with his characters. There's much more I'd like to tell you; I haven't even given you a complete list of the rosette chapters, but they are all there waiting for you to discover. All you have to do is visit your library or bookshop. You will have to take some time off from reading medical journals but I know that you work very hard and you deserve a treat. And, what is more, the experience could be more valuable profession-ally than the average postgraduate course. You may find, in a little while, that there are people in your surgery who are not unlike

Levin and Kitty and Stiva and Alexei Karenin. Doesn't that tearful mother with her three children remind you a little of Dolly? And what about that young woman with the pale face and the dark curly hair who's telling you about her drug habit and her lover who doesn't seem to care any more. And her thoughts about going down to the railway tracks …

Postscript by Alistair Stead

My friend John has entertainingly seduced you into reading Tolstoy's great novel by enacting something like a first-time reading. His is an appetite-whetting preface, whereas all I offer is a brief critical afterword, notes on things which might strike you once the first reading is over.

For instance, John alludes to the title: *Karenin* or *Karenina*? Only well into the book are you likely to consider that Anna *must* be Karenin (her husband's name, so his property), which poses, without settling, the whole moral question of the book. (Compare similar challenges in titles like *Madame Bovary* or *Mrs Dalloway*.) Should we condemn Anna for the dereliction of her duty as wife and mother, indicting perhaps a whole class of which Anna is only representative, or lament Anna's tragic bondage to Karenin, identifying an heroic vitality crushed by patriarchy?

Then there's the opening maxim: 'All happy families are alike but an unhappy family is unhappy after its own fashion.' As John asks, is it true? Does it matter? He speeds on to the story and the issue dangles. To begin the book with such a bold generalisation is intently provocative, soliciting 'how true' or 'on the contrary' (so Nabokov begins *Ada* with a parodic inversion of it). We may eventually reach a conclusion about the Oblonskys at least, but the large inclusiveness of the gesture foregrounds: (a) Tolstoy's focus on families themselves (the novel revolves around a few interlinked families, a family-tree approach revealing that Vronsky is the only major figure excluded, with his child by Anna becoming, legally, a Karenin) and on the moral value of family life, betrayed by the lovers; and (b) Tolstoy's focus on degrees of likeness and difference (the stuff of family life).

Tolstoy's greatness arguably lies in being simultaneously responsive to what *generally* happens and to the uniqueness of each person (Anna as type and autonomous being).

From the start, we move, characteristically, between Olympian long-shot and intimate close-up, portentous aphorism and succulent Oblonskyan incarnation. Within that maxim itself, 'happy'/'unhappy' initiates us into a massive counterpoint in the principal pairings (Anna and Vronsky, Levin and Kitty) and often ironic 'rhyming' of events. Tolstoy loves to thicken the texture by doubling, by parallelisms and antitheses, to impose, too, a remarkable sense of pattern even in so large a project. He valued 'that endless labyrinth of linkages', of ideas to be effected indirectly through words describing 'images, action, situations'. These are recognised consciously only after lengthy immersion in the book, evident in many repeated, slightly varied elements. Most obviously, there's the almost symmetrical placing of the scenes at the railway station – near the beginning as setting for the meeting of Anna and Vronsky, near the end for the suicide of Anna – a placing embedded in multiple references to train journeys and nightmare visions of death under the train's wheels. Less obvious, especially in translation where variations on *svet*, the Russian word for light, are hidden from view (a candle is *svecha*, a star is *svetilo*, etc.) is the cluster of light–fire symbols, recurrent but richly elaborated in the double climax. These register and set in balance Anna's gradual loss of radiance and clear-sightedness and Levin's groping toward enlightenment. They culminate for her, in the emblematic flickering of her candle flame on the eve of her death and in the flickering of her consciousness as she is annihilated by the train; for him in the rapture before starlight which constituted his moment of spiritual illumination – a moment, too, which may still, very humanly, flicker in its turn?

The text

Anna Karenin by Lev Tolstoy was first published in 1878. It is available in English in a number of paperback editions. The

English translation by Rosemary Edmonds was first published by Penguin Books Ltd, London in 1954. Extracts reproduced by permission of Penguin Books Ltd.

Further reading

Nabokov V (1982) *Lectures on Russian Literature*. Picador, London.

Thorlby A (1987) *Leo Tolstoy: Anna Karenina*. Landmarks of World Literature, Cambridge University Press, Cambridge.

Wilson AN (1989) *Tolstoy*. Penguin Books, Harmondsworth.

5

Mansfield Park

by Jane Austen

About the author

Jane Austen is one of the greatest, some would say *the* greatest of English novelists. Others find her appeal limited because she writes only about the small world in which she lived. As she said herself: 'three or four families in a country village is the very thing to work on'. The families are middle class and comfortably off (although they may have interesting poor relations as we shall see) and nothing very much happens, except the occasional dance or country walk. The chief characters are young women and their main preoccupation seems to be finding husbands. If you read Jane's books you soon discover that the girls are also concerned, like many fictional heroes, with the moral philosophical questions of how one should live and whether it is possible to do the right thing and still find your heart's desire. That sounds a bit solemn, so I must qualify it at once by saying that Jane sees life as essentially a comedy and delights in observing the absurdities of her characters and satirising their pretensions.

Who was Jane, and what was she like? A prim maiden lady, rather like your old English teacher? Never went anywhere, never got married. A detached observer of life who never really lived herself? And how did she learn to write so well?

She was born in 1775, the second daughter of a country clergyman. She had five brothers and one elder sister (Cassandra) of whom she was very fond. The only portrait we have of her is a quick sketch done by Cassandra, which shows a plump-faced, dark-eyed girl with a few wisps of curly hair escaping on to her forehead from underneath a mob cap. We know from letters and family memoirs that she was a normal teenager who enjoyed clothes, dancing, amateur theatricals and meeting boys. She also wrote stories and plays from an early age and had filled several notebooks with them by the time she was 16. Did she have a love life of her own? She was certainly very keen on a young man called Tom Lefroy, who came over from Ireland to stay with his uncle and aunt at Christmas 1795 and met the 21-year-old Jane at one of those country house dances for young people. There are many fond references to Tom in a letter which she wrote to Cassandra, and the feeling seems to have been mutual. Sadly, after the holidays, Tom Lefroy returned to Ireland where he met and married someone else and subsequently became Chief Justice of Ireland. He continued to be in Jane's thoughts for several years.

Thereafter, although she probably had several offers, none of the local boys she danced with seems to have made any impression on her heart. In December 1802, a young man with the striking name of Harris Bigg-Wither proposed to her in the library. Harris was the brother of one of Jane's friends, a shy boy with a stammer, whom she had known all her life. Everyone congratulated the couple but Jane spent a sleepless night and in the morning she told Harris that she couldn't marry him because, although she liked and respected him, she didn't love him. After that there were no more proposals and Jane just got on with her writing. Perhaps if she had become Mrs Bigg-Wither she would have had a rich and fulfilling family life (the woman Harris eventually married bore him 10 children). But would we have been deprived of *Pride and Prejudice, Emma* and *Mansfield Park*? Would we have had different books? It is hard to say. But I wanted you to know a bit about Jane's love life so you wouldn't think she was a dried-up old prune who experienced no emotions of her own. As to how she learned to write, that is amazing, because she never had any contact with other writers although she was an enthusiastic reader. She died in 1817, at the age of 41, after a long illness with weakness, back pain and recurrent fevers. Sir Zachary Cope, eminent physician and Austen fan, argued in an article in the *Lancet* in 1964 that she must have had Addison's disease, but this has since been disputed. She is buried in Winchester Cathedral where the epitaph on her tombstone omits to mention that she was a writer.

Mansfield Park

No, it's not an underground station near the outer limits of the Piccadilly line, it is one of Jane Austen's novels, the third to be published and probably the one I like best. When it came out, in 1813, most readers said they preferred *Pride and Prejudice*, which had more gaiety and sparkle. They found Mansfield's heroine, Fanny Price, to be rather a dim, self-righteous little girl very different from Elizabeth Bennett of *Pride and Prejudice*. And, to make things more difficult, *Mansfield Park* has an anti-heroine called Mary Crawford, whom some readers like a lot better – although I am not one of their number. The book provides plenty of entertainment as well as making you think (and feel) quite a lot. Jane never wrote anything else quite like it and – at the time I first wrote this chapter – it had not yet been turned into a film. I hoped that it never would be; or, if it was, that I would at least be allowed to direct it myself. I am sad to say that someone else has now filmed it and produced a rather inauthentic version in which Fanny is presented as a writer like Jane herself. Let us ignore that aberration and turn instead to the original.

This is how it begins:

> About thirty years ago, Miss Maria Ward of Huntingdon, with only seven thousand pounds had the good luck to captivate Sir Thomas Bertram, of Mansfield Park, in the county of Northampton, and to be thereby raised to the rank of a baronet's lady, with all the comforts and consequences of an handsome house and large income.

I know that some of you will have difficulty with the first chapter, because I did myself. It is written in a rather formal style and it is difficult to take in exactly what we are being told. It seems to be about some sisters getting married and some doing better for themselves than others. Then there's a discussion about whether her richer relatives can help the poorest sister by adopting her eldest girl and what effect this would have on the better-off children, and so on. It would be easy for your eyes to glide over the rather elaborate pompous diction of Sir Thomas and Mrs Norris (of whom more later) and for you to reach the end of Chapter 1 without really having retained any grasp of the careful setting of the scene which Jane prepared for you – in about 1811.

What is to be done? Well you could proceed straight to Chapter 2, which, since it introduces our heroine at the tender age of ten, will engage your empathies at once. If this cavalier treatment of chapters is unacceptable, I suggest that you take Chapter 1 slowly and try to construct a genogram, just as you would in the surgery if a nervous adolescent came to tell you about her family problems. The genogram will show that there are three Ward sisters. The middle one, Maria, marries the baronet Sir Thomas Bertram and moves in to the grand and spacious surroundings of Mansfield Park. The eldest (referred to by the convention of the time as simply 'Miss Ward') does rather less well for herself by marrying a poor clergyman, but his baronet brother-in-law provides him with a living, so they don't do so badly.

The youngest sister marries, 'to disoblige her family', a lieutenant of marines who is clearly an alcoholic no-hoper, and she proceeds to bear him nine children. Fanny Price, our little heroine, is the eldest daughter of this large family and the story really gets going when she is summarily removed from her family in Portsmouth to lighten her parents' burden – and brought to live among her socially superior relations, the Bertrams, at Mansfield Park.

The Bertrams have four children of their own, two boys and two girls, all a few years older than Fanny. How does our little waif appear to her new family? She is 'small of her age, with no glow of complexion, nor any other striking beauty; exceedingly timid and shy, and shrinking from notice'. In fact, she spends most of her time in the first few weeks crying to herself, as you might expect. Her aunt, Mrs Norris (the one who married the parson), is disgusted by this behaviour and thinks Fanny is not trying hard enough. Mrs Norris is a really obnoxious woman, perhaps the most self centred, non-empathic character in English literature (and one of the funniest). The others are less unpleasant, but as Jane tells us:

'Nobody meant to be unkind, but nobody put themselves out of their way to secure her comfort.' The two girls regard their little cousin with disdain when they find she has only two sashes and has never learnt French: you know how horrid little girls can be. As for the boys, Tom, the elder, is fairly indifferent to Fanny's existence, but the younger one, Edmund, is a kind, thoughtful boy who, we are relieved to find, is going to look after our little girl and be really nice to her. There is a tender scene in which Edmund discovers Fanny sitting at the foot of the stairs crying. He talks to her, asks her what's wrong, mentions that she might be missing her old home and then 'her increased sobs explained to him where the grievance lay'. Now some people find our Edmund a bit solemn and a bit of a prig, but there is no denying that he is a decent, sensitive lad who knows how to listen to a child in distress. He would make an excellent GP and is in fact going to be a country parson, which is the next best thing. Of course, Fanny comes to depend very much on Edmund's kindness and friendship and, as they both grow older, she naturally falls in love with him. This is far from what her uncle and aunt intended. They needn't have worried, because Fanny is and remains a timid little creature with very low self-esteem and almost zero expectations. She also gets tired very easily and I suspect that she doesn't eat much. I am really quite concerned about her. She doesn't see her own family for years and her depression goes unrecognised by everyone except Edmund (thank goodness he is there). However, she is very obliging to her aunts and is always willing to run errands and do little jobs around the house so that they soon find her indispensable.

This is all quite serious isn't it? More like Dickens than Jane Austen. No wonder early readers preferred *Pride and Prejudice*. But wait a little. The Austen fun and comedy are not to be excluded from *Mansfield Park* even if we do have a rather tragic heroine. And here come a couple of fresh characters, a brother and sister, new to the area, called Henry and Mary Crawford. The Crawfords are 'young people of fortune', who are used to the exciting social round of life in London. For some critics they represent the new-style middle-class English society which was beginning to be a threat to the quiet, settled ways of landed country families. The two Bertram girls, Maria and Julia, are both ready to submit to young Henry's debonair charm: which is really *not* the proper way for Maria to respond because she is supposed to be engaged to a local landowner and genial silly ass called Mr Rushworth. Mary Crawford takes a fancy to Edmund. She has some light-hearted, teasing conversations with him and poor, simple Edmund is quite smitten, although he can see that Mary is not really a serious person like he is. She is so frivolous about things like marriage and the clergy as a profession, and really her behaviour is quite immodest at times, but perhaps that's part of the attraction. Fanny, who is an observer of all these flirtatious activities, suffers terrible pangs of jealousy when she sees Edmund and Mary together – although she can scarcely admit even to herself that she could ever be a serious candidate. When Edmund borrows back the horse he has given to Fanny so that Mary can have daily rides, she gives it up gracefully – only too pleased to be able to help. But the sight of Edmund and Mary riding together is exquisitely painful for her – especially when he appears to be holding her hand. Fanny spends the rest of the day cutting roses in the hot sun and running between Mansfield and Aunt Norris's house. She develops a headache and is almost fainting when Edmund returns. Her aunts are inclined to blame it on the heat, but Edmund is full of remorse at neglecting his little cousin. And we doctors know a psychosomatic illness when it is thrust in our faces.

The next adventure is an excursion by all the young people to visit Maria's fiancé's country house at Sotherton. This provides all sorts of opportunities for romantic walks in the woods by our inappropriately flirting couples: Mary Crawford manages to get Edmund to herself, leaving Fanny resting on a park bench; and Maria and Henry give Maria's fiancé the slip by sending him back to the house for a key to a gate to the woods, while they slip through a gap in the hedge. Again, our Fanny has to be the helpless observer of these antics, which distress her both personally and because she has such a strong moral instinct. (I call it an instinct because it is not clear where she gets it from.) When they finally get back to Mansfield, Aunt Norris, so often the vehicle for the author's irony, says to her niece: 'Well, Fanny, this has been a fine day for you, upon my word! ... Nothing but pleasure from beginning to end!'

Now comes an important conversation between Edmund, Mary Crawford and Fanny. They are discussing Edmund's intention to become ordained and take up the profession of country parson. (Jane Austen told someone when she was planning *Mansfield Park* that her next novel was to be about 'ordination'. No doubt he was completely mystified.) Mary's view is that this is no sort of job for a Mansfield boy. As far as she is concerned, your typical clergyman is just an idle slob who 'has the best intention of doing nothing all the rest of his days but eat, drink and grow fat … A clergyman has nothing to do but to be slovenly and selfish – read the newspaper, watch the weather, and quarrel with his wife. His curate does all the work and the business of his own life is to dine.' This rather biased view derives from her experience of her brother-in-law Dr Grant and, as Fanny points out, in an unusually bold speech for her, is not based on evidence from a representative sample. This conversation is one of a series threaded throughout the story in which Mary tries to get Edmund to give up his ambition to be a country vicar and be more cool. Fanny is usually on hand to support the idea of the church as a noble and satisfying vocation (and the kind of life she would be only too happy to share, given half a chance and if she dared even think about it).

Now we come to the amateur theatricals episode, one of Jane's most brilliant set pieces and perhaps the most entertaining part of a book crowded with incidents. While Sir Thomas is away looking after his business interests in Antigua (slave trade? Very possibly, but we are not going into that at present), the young people decide it would be great fun to put on a play. This is suggested by a friend called Mr Yates, who has just come from staying with some other country house thespians whose play was rudely interrupted (as this one will be too). Our young people take up the idea of a play with great enthusiasm – all except Edmund and Fanny, who are dead against it. Why, for heaven's sake? What can be wrong with a bit of amateur acting? What are they afraid of? This is a question that has been much discussed by the critics ever since the book was written. Amateur theatricals were very popular at the time and Jane was known to enjoy them herself. But there are a number of problems with this particular production for our hero and heroine, as we soon discover.

First of all, father is away and everyone feels in their bones that if he knew, he wouldn't like it. Especially if it means moving the furniture about and turning his dressing room into a green room. Then there is the play they have chosen, a real one called *Lovers' Vows*. I don't have space to give you the plot in detail. I'll just tell you that, rather like the walk in the woods, it provides opportunities for some rather sexy dalliance between boy and girl. Maria Bertram takes one of these parts, coupled with Henry Crawford (although she's still engaged to Rushworth), and smiling, sexy Mary Crawford lands, without much difficulty, the part of an eagerly amorous young woman. At first there is some uncertainty about who is to play the part of her lover, the Reverend Mr Anhalt (oh, no! Not a lecherous clergyman). '"Who is to be Anhalt?"' (asks Mary innocently). '"What gentleman among you am I to have the pleasure of making love to?" For a moment no one spoke …'. (I'm not a bit surprised – that's quite a Mae West of a line even if it didn't have quite the same meaning in 1814 as it would now.) Yes, you're right. Edmund ends up doing it, because he can't bear the thought of an outsider being brought in and possibly getting off with Mary in real life.

He asks poor Fanny to support him in this decision and, to her credit, she won't. She also refuses to act even a small part herself: 'I could not act any thing if you were to give me the world.' I think one of the points Jane is making is that some people (like Fanny) can only be themselves. While Mary and Henry, who take to theatricals like ducks to water, are acting most of the time, always concerned to give a stylish performance. But Fanny, although she won't act, is unable to break the habit of being everyone's little helper. She teaches everyone their lines (Mr Rushworth, a great comic creation and a true *schlemiel*, is very proud that his part has 42 speeches, although he seems incapable of remembering any of them). She even has to endure the misery of hearing Edmund and Mary enthusiastically rehearse their love scene, since they have both sought her out separately for some coaching.

Only sister Julia has been excluded from the play, having been bumped out of the two main parts by the scheming Henry. However, she does get the most dramatic line in the novel: just as the players are about to begin their first full rehearsal on stage,

Julia throws open the door and 'with a face all aghast, exclaimed, "My father is come! He is in the hall at this moment."'

And that's the last we see of *Lover's Vows*, but some wonderfully comic scenes are to follow as Sir Thomas gradually realises what has been going on in his house and – as we predicted – is not at all pleased. At one point he goes to his dressing room, finds the bookcase moved and the door to the billiard room (now the stage) open. He goes through to find himself on the stage opposite a ranting young man in a pink satin cloak (Mr Yates as a fictional Baron Wildenhaim). Ironic Jane describes it as Sir Thomas's 'first appearance on any stage'. There is a lovely description of Mr Yates gradually realising what has happened and transforming himself from a ranting Baron, back into a well-bred young man. A truly theatrical scene!

We are not even halfway through the book yet, so I shall have to quicken my pace and just give you an outline of what follows. But by the time you have got this far, you will be well engrossed in the story and fully adapted to Jane's prose style which, once you are used to its gentle rhythms, is delightful to read.

The next major event is that Henry begins to notice Fanny and decides it would be fun to see if he can make her fall in love with him. She is about 19 by now and beginning to blossom, especially when her favourite brother, William, a young sailor, comes to visit. We had almost forgotten that she had any family of her own. It is really a pleasure to see her so happy and lively in his company. (Jane, too, had brothers in the navy and knew a lot about the life of serving naval officers.) Henry tells his sister that he only wants to make 'a small hole in Fanny Price's heart. I will not do her any harm, dear little soul! I only want her to look kindly on me, to give me smiles as well as blushes, to keep a chair for me by herself wherever we are, and be all animated when I take it and talk to her … and feel when I go away that she shall never be happy again. I want nothing more.' 'Moderation itself!' says his sister. And we think: 'what a swine!'

But, I'm happy to say, the plan unravels rapidly. Fanny rejects him, while being grateful for his kindness to William. Then he *really* falls in love with her (perhaps for the first time in his life). He woos the frightened girl desperately, abetted by letters from his sister urging her to take pity on him. We wonder if Bad Henry is going to turn over a new moral leaf and be reborn as Good Henry. The family at Mansfield are, of course, outraged that a little nobody like Fanny Price can have the nerve to refuse such a good offer. 'What does she want?' they ask themselves. There is a magnificent scene in the schoolroom (Fanny's special private place where she retires to lick her wounds) in which Sir Thomas attempts to persuade her to accept Henry. Even Edmund (still captivated by Mary but worried about her morals) thinks she should give in. But Fanny is obdurate. Good for Fanny. Jane Austen, we know, thought nobody should enter a loveless marriage; she undoubtedly remained single herself because of this strong conviction. So don't be deceived by all that apparently cynical stuff about people marrying for money.

However, Sir Thomas still hopes that Fanny will change her mind. He hatches a plan to send her back to Portsmouth to stay with her parents and siblings for a while. He reasons to himself that a shock reacquaintance with poverty will make her really appreciate the comfort of a middle-class lifestyle – and the advantages of agreeing to marry Henry Crawford. The opportunity comes when Fanny's brother William has a spot of leave from the navy and pays another visit to his sister at Mansfield. When the time comes for him to rejoin his ship, Fanny travels down with him to Portsmouth and spends a couple of months with her mother and father and numerous younger siblings. She is rather appalled by their rough manners. The house is not only cramped, it is terribly disorganised and everyone is so noisy! Fanny longs to be back in the calm and comfort of Mansfield. However, she can see that sister Susan (15) has some potential and decides to take her education in hand. Our heroine realises that she has come a long way since she left Portsmouth and that there is no way in which she could possibly merge back into her family of origin.

What happens in the end? I'm not going to tell you any more, except that Fanny emerges a happy and contented young lady. Some people may find her unsympathetic and unbelievably virtuous, but I don't agree. From the moment we meet her in Chapter 2 as a tearful ten-year-old snatched from her mother, she is a warm, utterly human and, for me, completely real character. She is full of feeling and my heart keeps perfect time with hers as it flutters away in agitation and (occasionally) joy. In *Mansfield Park*, Jane Austen wanted to achieve something more serious than *Pride and Prejudice* without losing too much of the sparkle of her earlier style. We can learn a lot about human relationships and experience deeply satisfying feelings from this book, as well as being richly entertained by the comedy. It waits, patiently, on a shelf in a bookshop near you. Go get it.

The text

Mansfield Park (1814) by Jane Austen is available in the Penguin Classics series, with an introduction by Tony Tanner.

Further reading

Tomalin C (1997) *Jane Austen, A Life*. Viking, London.

6

Wuthering Heights

by Emily Jane Brontë

About the author

Once upon a time there were three little girls called Charlotte, Emily and Anne, who loved to sit around the kitchen table writing stories and poems. They lived with their father, the curate, in a large vicarage in a small town high up on the Yorkshire moors. They had a brother called Branwell, who also enjoyed writing but unfortunately took to drink. Their mother and two older sisters had died tragically young from tuberculosis. When the three remaining sisters reached their twenties, they started writing novels under the supervision of the eldest sister, Charlotte, who was determined to get them published even if she had to pretend they were all men. Emily, the middle sister, only produced one novel, but it was brilliant. It is such a strange and disturbing story that it has a unique place in English literature. Since it was first published in 1847 there has never been anything quite like it and we still don't understand how or why Emily wrote it.

Even her sister Charlotte (whose own books were quite disturbing) felt obliged to issue a health warning for prospective readers. She, and everyone who has read the book since, have been particularly worried by the character of Heathcliff, who is both the hero and demonic villain of *Wuthering Heights*. 'Whether it is right or advisable to create things like Heathcliff, I do not know' (wrote Charlotte in her preface to the first edition) 'I scarcely think it is.'

But wait a moment, some of you will say. Isn't Heathcliff the tall, dark, passionate, romantic hero played in the old black-and-white film by Laurence Olivier? And isn't it a love story set in beautiful northern English hill country so familiar to us from the James Herriott country vet stories and the Catherine Cookson serials on TV?

Well, the Yorkshire of Emily's imagination isn't quite like that. The landscape may be the same but it is painted in darker colours and the weather can be a good deal rougher. As for the characters, they make you wonder, as her sister no doubt did, how a well brought up young woman could conceive of such people. By now, if you haven't read the book (or not since you were at school) you must be getting impatient for evidence. So let us open Emily's story at page one and begin.

The story begins

Even the first chapter is a little unsettling. It begins with the date '1801', so we know where we are in time, more or less, but that's about all. The story is told in the first person by a Mr Lockwood, who appears to be an amiable, upper-class young man, probably not long down from university. He has been disappointed in love and has fled from society to the remote desolation of Yorkshire, where he has apparently rented a house on or near the moors. As the story opens he is paying a call on his landlord, who is none other than Mr Heathcliff and who lives in another house, higher up on the fells, called Wuthering Heights.

Wuthering Heights, as you might expect from the name, is a massive, rather forbidding structure, built to withstand the howling winds and winter snows of the moorland tops and not offering much comfort apart from a blazing fire. Mr Heathcliff, the owner, is a grim fellow with 'black eyes drawn so suspiciously under their brows', and he doesn't go out of his way to make his young visitor feel at ease. Nevertheless, he does invite Lockwood in and rather grudgingly offers him a glass of wine. While Heathcliff is down in the cellar with his gratuitously offensive manservant, Joseph, Lockwood tries to make friends with the snarling dogs and is attacked for his pains. However, things settle down, they have a chat over their wine and Lockwood departs for his own house determined to visit again the next day.

In Chapter 2, we learn a bit more about the lie of the land. Lockwood is staying at Heathcliff's other house, which lies four miles down the hill from Wuthering Heights. The Grange is a much more gracious and comfortable place than the forbidding Heights and is really more of a stately home, enclosed in its own park. So why does Heathcliff own two houses and choose to live in the less comfortable one? Have patience! One of the joys of reading is the gradual clarification of mysteries.

The next day, despite the wintry weather, Lockwood decides to set out once again 'wading through heath and mud' to visit Wuthering Heights. Once again he has a rather rough reception, this time from Joseph, who shouts at him in Yorkshire dialect. (Joseph, who is a half-crazed, misanthropic, religious zealot, speaks entirely in dialect, which is presumably an accurate rendering of how Yorkshire farm labourers spoke in the 1840s (or earlier) but is only partly comprehensible even if, like me, you were born in Yorkshire only 20 miles from the Brontë home in Haworth.)

This time we meet two other members of the household, a young man and a young woman. Lockwood has great difficulty in working out the relationship of these two to the stern Mr Heathcliff and keeps embarrassing himself by getting it wrong. We readers are equally puzzled and are quite glad to have Lockwood (to whom we helplessly cling in this strange, already sinister place) make the mistakes instead of us. Let me introduce the newcomers.

The young woman is slender, fair and beautiful and, as we shall discover, only 17. She is called Cathy and Lockwood is immediately attracted to her, although his fantasies come to nothing (and just as well). Like everyone at the Heights she is not exactly welcoming and is reluctant even to let him have a cup of tea. At first Lockwood takes her for Heathcliff's wife, but she turns out to be his daughter-in-law. What about the surly, shabbily dressed young man then, is he the husband of the fair girl and Mr Heathcliff's son? Wrong again. This conjecture is greeted with derision by Heathcliff and rage by the young man who goes red in the face and growls that his name is Hareton Earnshaw 'and I'd counsel you to respect it!'. The three members of this dysfunctional family (four if we include the servant Joseph) all seem to hate each other and they are really not nice to be with for a genteel outsider like Lockwood. But now things get even worse for the poor chap. After an uncomfortable meal he tries to head for home. But it is snowing heavily and the road is covered. Will anyone guide him across the moors? There are no offers and when, in desperation, he tries to borrow the lantern, he is accused of stealing it by Joseph, who sets the dogs on him. Poor Lockwood has a terrible fright and his nose starts bleeding. At last he is rescued by the housekeeper, who appears suddenly with a glass of water which she throws down his neck (presumably to cure the epistaxis). He is led inside, given a glass of brandy and at last offered a bed for the night.

Sleeping over at Wuthering Heights

Chapter 3 describes Lockwood's overnight experience at Wuthering Heights and it is rather scary. He goes to bed in a kind of cupboard and, unable to sleep, starts idly leafing through a pile of books on the windowsill (the way you do when you stay in someone else's bedroom). He finds that the books belong to someone called Catherine Earnshaw, but not the young Catherine downstairs as the flyleaf is dated 25 years earlier. This Catherine has the habit of using her books as a diary by writing between the lines of the printed text (something the little Brontë girls used to do as well). He starts to read, and Emily very cleverly shifts the narration from Lockwood to the mysterious Catherine who takes over her own story for a while. It is like a cinematic flashback introduced by a dissolve as we see Lockwood beginning to decipher the words ...

Now we are in the world of the elder Catherine's childhood on 'An awful Sunday ...'. We are still at Wuthering Heights. Catherine's father is away and she is in the care of her elder brother and his wife. Joseph is still around, ranting at everyone and invoking the scriptures in his hideous dialect. And Catherine has a playmate with whom she is obviously very close (or 'thick' as Emily would say), a boy called Heathcliff! The two kids feel oppressed by the adults and plan to escape to the moors together.

At this point Lockwood dozes off and the vision of Catherine's childhood fades. Lockwood dreams, at first of being in chapel and enduring a long, tedious sermon. Then he seems to hear a tapping sound apparently due to a fir tree branch knocking at the window in the ever-present wind and snow which surround Wuthering Heights. Unable to open the window, he knocks out the glass to stop the tapping, puts an arm through and finds his fingers 'closed on the fingers of a little ice-cold hand!'

The owner of the hand is a young girl who says her name is Catherine (naturally). She has lost her way on the moors and wants to come in. Lockwood is terrified and tries to withdraw but Catherine (or is it her ghost?) clutches on to his arm and won't let go. In the first of a number of examples of rather shocking cruelty in the book, Lockwood rubs the girl's bare arm against the broken glass 'till the blood ran down and soaked the bedclothes'. By now, we readers are sitting bolt upright with beads of cold sweat on our foreheads. What the hell is going to happen next? We didn't know this was going to be a scary ghost story. Well I did warn you at the beginning – and it is only partly a ghost story. There is much more besides.

The spectral Cathy finally lets go of Lockwood's arm but continues to moan at the window. He starts yelling in terror and awakes Mr Heathcliff, who comes in and demands to know what the noise is about. When Lockwood tells him about his dream Heathcliff is stunned and appears to be struggling with violent emotions. After dismissing Lockwood from the bedroom he wrenches open the window and calls desperately for Cathy, 'my heart's darling', to come to him. This is a different Heathcliff, overcome with grief for his lost love. For the first time our attitude to him softens a little. We can even forgive some of his ill temper and bad manners. And we desperately need to know what happened to separate the childhood sweethearts.

At this point I think we also desperately need a genogram or family tree to help us sort out some of the relationships in and around Wuthering Heights. In my Penguin edition, the introduction includes a very useful family tree, complete with dates of births, marriages and deaths. Further help is at hand from the next narrator who now takes over for most of the rest of the book.

Nelly Dean takes over the story

Lockwood arrives back at the Grange more dead than alive, having followed his scary night by getting lost in the snow on the last stages of his journey home (Heathcliff recovered himself sufficiently to escort him halfway back – one of our hero's rare examples of ordinary human generosity). He needs a lengthy rest at home before venturing out again and he takes the opportunity of asking the housekeeper, Ellen (Nelly) Dean, to tell him something of the history of the strange folk at Wuthering Heights. This she proceeds to do and most of what we hear from now on is in the words of Nelly Dean, as related to Mr Lockwood.

Once again, Emily uses her 'dissolve to flashback' technique and we soon forget that we are listening to the middle-aged Nelly recounting her memories. Instead we are translated back with her to when she herself was a child of about 12, the daughter of a house servant at Wuthering Heights and allowed to play with the children of the master and mistress.

One day (recalls Nelly) Mr Earnshaw, the father of her play-mate Hindley Earnshaw (14) and his little sister Catherine (6), returns to Wuthering Heights from a trip to Liverpool bringing with him 'a dirty ragged, black-haired child' whom he had found starving and homeless and decided to adopt. They name him Heathcliff (after a child who died), they give him a good wash and he becomes part of the household, although never accepted as a full member of the family. Nobody likes him much except the old master and, of course, little Cathy. He is only a year older than her and the two children soon become firm friends and allies. He also bonds with Nelly when she nurses him through the measles. But he soon shows the hard, ruthless strain in his character in his dealings with his older foster brother Hindley, whom he forces to exchange horses with him when his own goes lame.

Time goes on; the children grow up, and Cathy and Heathcliff become even closer. Catherine is mischievous and her strict father is fairly cool towards her. Hindley doesn't much like his little sister either and so Heathcliff is her only friend. When the parents die they are left to the care of brother Hindley and his wife Frances. She is quite a reasonable person (there aren't all that many in *Wuthering Heights* so it's quite striking when you meet one), but he is determined to prevent his little foster brother Heathcliff from getting any sort of education or becoming a gentleman. And he certainly doesn't mean him to get any share of the property. So Heathcliff and Catherine reach adolescence as rather a wild pair, forever running off to the moors together and sharing secrets. One day they visit the big house in the valley (Thrushcross Grange. Remember?) and peer through the windows at the splendid carpets and furniture inside. The two ragged children are spotted and the dogs are set on them. Heathcliff escapes but Cathy is bitten on the leg and gets captured. Once inside the house, the Linton family (who live there) realise who she is – the daughter of those peculiar but just about respectable people who live up the top of the moor. She stays on a few weeks to recover from her wound and gets to know the Linton children, Edgar and Isabella. When she returns to Wuthering Heights she is smartly dressed and looks a real lady – to the dismay of Heathcliff, who is scolded for touching her white dress and leaving his dirty paw marks on it.

This is the beginning of a friendship between Catherine and young Edgar Linton, who starts to pay calls on her at Wuthering Heights. Cathy's family try to keep Heathcliff out of sight lest his scruffy, already slightly threatening, appearance frightens the rather dainty Edgar and his sister. Heathcliff smoulders with jealousy, although Cathy repeatedly assures him that she still cares for him. Edgar makes an ill-judged observation about the length of Heathcliff's hair and gets a tureen of hot apple sauce thrown in his face. When Heathcliff is summarily punished, Cathy flies to his defence and admonishes Edgar for upsetting him in the first place.

Nelly continues to relate her history of life at the Heights, where the emotional tempests within its thick walls perfectly match the stormy weather that rages outside. Cathy, at 16, is 'the queen of the country-side' according to Nelly, and 'a haughty headstrong creature'. She continues to be friendly with Edgar, who soon falls in love with her – to Heathcliff's dismay. Meanwhile elder brother Hindley and sister-in-law Frances have had a child, a boy called Hareton. Frances dies in childbirth and her husband takes seriously to drink. Nelly, who is still only 22, takes over baby Hareton's upbringing and is now the only sane member of the family. Heathcliff broods hatefully about how he can take his revenge on his adoptive family.

A pause for reflection

At this point, you might be wondering why Emily Brontë peopled her story with such savage and spiteful characters. Was her home life at the parsonage like this? On the whole, no, even if brother Branwell came home the worse for drink now and then. It is worth remembering that all the Brontë children lived parallel lives in two fantasy worlds, which they talked and wrote about constantly. Emily and Anne shared an imaginary world called Gondal, which had a landscape not unlike Yorkshire but was full of proud, passionate princes and princesses. They wrote lots of stories in little notebooks, but sadly these have not survived and we only know about Gondal from a few references in poems and letters. In one famous diary page that has survived, the 16-year-old Emily describes an ordinary scene in the Brontë kitchen with Papa coming in and giving Branwell a letter. Then in the next sentence she says: 'The Gondals are discovering the interior of Gaaldine'. So fantasy and reality were very much side by side in Emily's mind and Wuthering Heights may be located as much in Gondal as in Yorkshire.

Cathy opens her heart to Nelly

On with the story. In Chapter 9, the 17-year-old Cathy goes to Nelly for some counselling about whether she should marry young Edgar Linton. She quickly reveals that she has accepted and will marry him, but she wants Nelly to tell her whether she has done the right thing. Nelly handles this tricky presentation quite skilfully and encourages Cathy to reflect on her feelings. She says she loves Edgar because he is handsome and is going to be rich and because he loves her. Not good enough, says Nelly. And because 'I shall enjoy being the greatest woman in the neighbourhood'. So what's the problem? Where is the obstacle? asks Nelly. 'Here! and here!' cries Catherine, striking one hand on her forehead and the other on her breast. 'In whichever place the soul lives – in my soul and in my heart, I'm convinced that I'm wrong!' And in a poetic and moving series of speeches she tells Nelly that Heathcliff is her true love: 'Whatever our souls are made of, his and mine are the same and Linton's is as different as a moonbeam from lightning, or frost from fire.' Unhappily she can't marry him now because brother Hindley has 'brought him so low' and it would degrade her to have him as a husband. Nevertheless, she does not intend to be parted from Heathcliff even though she's married to Edgar. In a famous and memorable passage, she compares her feelings about her two men to the ever-present landscape around Wuthering Heights:

> My love for Linton is like the foliage in the woods. Time will change it, I'm well aware, as winter changes the trees. My love for Heathcliff resembles the eternal rocks beneath – a source of little visible delight, but necessary. Nelly I am Heathcliff – he's always, always in my mind …

It is not a very conventional or Christian view of marriage to come from the pen of a respectable clergyman's daughter, is it? No wonder early Victorian readers were shocked. Even today it makes you wonder whether this sort of arrangement is really a good idea. Heathcliff certainly doesn't approve. He has been skulking in the background, listening, but unfortunately he arrived too late to hear Cathy's declaration of her love for him. Nelly sees him silently depart when he hears Cathy say it would 'degrade' her to marry Heathcliff now. In fact, Heathcliff is so upset that he disappears and, although Cathy waits and watches for him outside in the pouring rain for half the night and nearly catches her death of a fever (pneumonia?), we don't see him again for several years.

The return of Heathcliff

And so, Catherine and Edgar are married and live together at Thrushcross Grange. Nelly moves in to look after them (and because Emily needs her on hand to continue the narrative). One September evening Nelly is returning from the orchard with a basket of apples when she hears a voice calling her name. In the light of the full moon she sees a tall, dark figure standing in the porch. Heathcliff is back! He has used his time away to make himself over as a gentleman and is now well-dressed, distinguished-looking and well-spoken. There is something about this sudden appearance by moonlight which reminds me of another tall, handsome, sinister figure I've seen in a film. No, it's not Laurence Olivier, who can it be? I know, it's Christopher Lee playing the part of Count Dracula, the vampire in the brilliant 1958 Hammer film directed by Terence Fisher. Lee's Dracula is always the perfect gent and beautifully turned out in black cloak with scarlet lining. But when he bares his canines in a snarl of blood lust, by heaven, you know with whom or what you are dealing. And, on at least one occasion in the novel, one of the other characters wonders if Heathcliff is a human or a vampire? Heathcliff is now driven by two motivating forces: to be with Cathy once again and to destroy and dispossess just about everyone else (except Nelly for whom he retains a soft spot – remember the measles?)

Rather reluctantly Nelly allows him into the house and he and Cathy are joyfully reunited. Edgar is not too happy about the sudden reappearance of this old friend of the family, especially when he goes in for urgent, passionate, low-voiced conversations with Cathy. But he seems to tolerate Heathcliff's visits up to a point. Meanwhile Heathcliff is also pursuing his revenge on the two families who have excluded and spurned him. He goes up to Wuthering Heights and joins in Hindley's regular card games, gradually winning all his money. In another plan, he encourages Edgar's sister, Isabella, to become infatuated with him. His aim is to marry her and get a stake in the Linton property, and to bankrupt Hindley so that he will eventually become the owner of Wuthering Heights instead of Hindley's son. Both plans are carried out with cold, ruthless determination and both succeed.

Now Cathy and Heathcliff start quarrelling. Nelly is fearful for her mistress's emotional stability and sends for her husband. Edgar tries to throw Heathcliff out, although his wife shouts at him to leave them alone. He manages to wind Heathcliff with a blow to the throat and then rushes out to get reinforcements. Heathcliff at first refuses to go: 'I'll crush his ribs in like a rotten hazelnut', he roars, and makes it clear that it is only because Cathy places some value on her husband's life that he refrains from murdering him. ('The moment her regard ceased, I would have torn his heart out and drunk his blood!') Finally he smashes the door lock with a poker and storms off. Cathy rages at Nelly and Edgar and collapses in a fit which seems to be hysterical.

She retires to her bedroom for three days. Then she enters a kind of delirious state in which she dreams she is a child again, roaming the moors with Heathcliff. She alternately dreams and rants at everybody who tries to help, including her hapless husband. Clearly it is time the doctor was sent for and fortunately Nelly is able to intercept him in the High Street in between visits. Dr Kenneth (as he is called) seems to spend all his time doing house calls – I don't think he has a surgery. And as the pace of events builds up in Wuthering Heights he seems to be constantly hurrying between the Heights and the Grange uttering dire warnings about what will happen if his patients continue their reckless ways. Like a good country GP he is alert for the psychosocial factors in his patients' problems and he asks Nelly: 'What has there been to do at the Grange? We've odd reports up here. A stout hearty lass like Catherine does not fall ill for a trifle … How did it begin?' And so Nelly tells him about Heathcliff's visits. Having examined Catherine, he pronounces that she is to have around her 'perfect peace and tranquillity'. This is good health promotion advice, no doubt, but hopelessly unrealistic in a Brontë novel.

A birth and a death

Catherine recovers sufficiently to sit around the house but she has lost all her former strength and spirit. Her face is pale and her eyes have a faraway look. Heathcliff visits her one more time and, in the most passionate love scene in the book, they smother each other with kisses, tears and reproaches. She says he has killed her and he says she is to blame for murdering herself. Once again they are interrupted by the return of Edgar from church. Catherine faints away and Heathcliff retires to the garden to await events. The beginning of the next chapter tells us that on that same night Catherine gives birth to a daughter. There are no descriptions of sex in the book and you wouldn't expect any, would you? But you can't help noticing the way passionate embraces lead to sudden childbirth. Unhappily, the birth is too much for Cathy and she expires two hours later. The daughter is, of course, the younger Catherine. When Nelly tells him of her death, Heathcliff is inconsolable. He bangs his head against a gnarled oak tree and howls. He curses her for deserting him ('may she wake in torment!'). He calls upon her to haunt him and cries that he cannot live without her. Once again we have a pang of compassion for the monster. But this is soon dissipated as he continues with his plans for the ruination of the Lintons and Earnshaws.

What does he do? He carries off Edgar's sister, Isabella, marries her and then imprisons her in Wuthering Heights, where he treats her quite brutally. He has a fight with the drunken Hindley who dies shortly afterwards in mysterious circumstances without the doctor being called in. Hmm. Very suspicious. Hindley dies deeply in debt with Heathcliff his major creditor, so Heathcliff is now the *de facto* owner of Wuthering Heights. We also learn that Isabella has born him a son (called Linton), a sickly boy whom his father despises. Heathcliff's plan now is to mate Linton with the younger Catherine and thus gain control of both the heirs of the Linton family.

Cathy's daughter meets Heathcliff's son

Nelly's story now shifts to the childhood of the younger Catherine, of whom she is very fond. Once again Nelly is left in charge of the baby as parents drop dead all around her. However, Catherine's father, Edgar, is still alive and they have a good relationship, so she has quite a happy Heathcliff-free childhood at Thrushcross

Grange. Nelly's story moves on and the next chapter introduces a new character, Heathcliff's son. Little Linton Heathcliff is about the same age as Cathy Jr. And, when she first meets her cousin, Cathy is delighted with him. He's so pretty, with his pale, delicate skin and fair hair, she can't wait to play with him. And when they both get into their teens she has a secret romance with him, exchanging clandestine love letters. Heathcliff encourages them, of course, because it's all part of his plan that they should marry. He has nothing but contempt for his weedy little son ('I'm bitterly disappointed with the whey-faced, whining wretch!' he says to Nelly).

Now at first we are led to hope that young Cathy is going to help cousin Linton grow up, stiffen his sinews a little and stop whinging. Unfortunately, he's not only self-pitying, he's actually quite mean and spiteful. I find this part of the book quite distressing to read, as poor Cathy keeps trying to forge a proper relationship with Linton of whom she is genuinely fond. But as Linton gets physically weaker – he probably has tuberculosis like so many of the people in *Wuthering Heights* – his character deteriorates as well. Finally, Heathcliff uses Linton as a bait to lure Cathy to Wuthering Heights and then keeps her there as a prisoner in order to get her married to Linton before he dies. When Cathy tries to get the key off him (by biting his hand), Heathcliff gives her 'a shower of terrific slaps round the head'. Heathcliff has really become a monster, a wolfish man with snarling canines who hates his own kith and kin. What are we to make of him? What has happened to the passionate young man who was so full of love for Catherine Earnshaw, Cathy's mother? And what will happen to poor little Cathy, destined for a forcible marriage to the vampire's unwholesome offspring?

A happy ending?

Happily, if we stick with Cathy through this terrible phase of her story, we find things beginning to come right for her. She does have to marry Linton but his health goes rapidly downhill within weeks. Heathcliff refuses to get the doctor for his son because, he says, 'his life is not worth a farthing and I won't spend a farthing on him'. So Cathy becomes a widow and lives on at the Heights with Heathcliff – and with her other cousin, Hareton, whose father has been dispossessed and possibly murdered by Heathcliff. Hareton is resentful and rude to Cathy at first, but she is attracted to him and gradually wins him round and teaches him to read (he has been deliberately deprived of education by Heathcliff). So Cathy and Hareton get married and there is a happy ending, at least for them. But what about Heathcliff? Our friend Mr Lockwood returns to Yorkshire after a year's interval and seeks out Nelly to find out what has been happening in his absence. To his surprise, he learns that Heathcliff is dead. Nelly tells him that Heathcliff was unable to prevent Cathy and Hareton becoming fond of each other. Much of the bitterness and brutality seemed to have drained out of him. Possibly the sight of Hareton and the younger Catherine remind him of his own younger self and Catherine's mother. 'Nelly, there is a strange change approaching' he tells his old nurse, 'I'm in its shadow at present – I take so little interest in my daily life I hardly remember to eat and drink.' He spends a night out in the open, then comes back in the morning and retires to his room, refusing food. Good-hearted Nelly is quite concerned at his deterioration and his macabre appearance: 'Is he a ghoul or a vampire?' she muses. 'I had read of such hideous incarnate demons. And then, I set myself to reflect how I had tended him in infancy; and watched him grow to youth; and followed him through his whole course; and what absurd nonsense it was to yield to that sense of horror.' Good old Nelly: she is so down-to-earth and sensible.

Now I'm feeling sorry for Heathcliff again, although he still gives me the creeps when he bares his wolfish teeth. Shortly afterwards, Nelly finds him dead in his bed, but Dr Kenneth is unable to pronounce on the cause. He is buried – as he had wished – beside his Cathy, with Edgar on her other side. We already know that he has bribed the sexton to remove the sides of the two coffins separating him from Cathy so that their remains can be united in death. The three graves lie 'on the slope next the moor' and we are not surprised to hear that some of the locals have seen his ghost walking on the moors – and one terrified little boy claims to have seen him with a woman! Lockwood, as ever, finds such things hard to imagine.

And so we reach the end of this strange and wonderful book – a landmark in English literature, which stands out like a craggy monolith in the middle of the Yorkshire moors.

I hope you will read *Wuthering Heights* and experience both the agony and the ecstasy. And next time you are in Yorkshire, go and visit the Brontë Parsonage in Haworth. As you step out from the house on to the springy turf of Haworth Moor it is easy to believe that Wuthering Heights is just over the brow of the hill and that Heathcliff's spirit is brooding nearby. This is the house where those three little girls grew up, wove their fantasies, wrote their books – and succumbed, tragically young, to the dreaded tubercle bacillus. Emily refused to take any medicine throughout her final illness and would not allow anyone to send for the doctor until the last day of her life. Only then was Dr Wheelhouse allowed to come – and of course there was nothing he could do. No Rifinah in those days. Emily died in December 1848, just over a year after the publication of *Wuthering Heights*, at the age of 30. She was buried in the family vault in Haworth Churchyard. The funeral cortège was led by her bereaved father and her faithful dog, Keeper, walking side by side.

The text

Wuthering Heights (1847) by Emily Jane Brontë is available in the Penguin Classics series, with an introduction by David Daiches.

Further reading

Barker J (1994) *The Brontës*. Weidenfeld and Nicholson, London (paperback edition 1995). This is an excellent biography of the Brontë family.

7

Ulysses

by James Joyce

I have another big one for you now: 933 pages in the Penguin edition, and it comes with a fearsome reputation for being difficult. Have no fear. Would I offer you something unreadable? Certainly not. And, furthermore, it is another of my favourite, indispensable bedside books. Comparable to, well, Plumtree's potted meat. Plumtree's what? One of the joys of reading *Ulysses* is that you collect hundreds of little phrases, rhymes, puns, jokes, etc., which become treasured additions to the bric-à-brac on the mental mantelpiece. Some of them come from advertisements that were to be found in Dublin newspapers on 16 June 1904, which is where and when the story takes place. For example:

> *What is home without*
> *Plumtree's potted meat?*
> *Incomplete.*
> *With it an abode of bliss.*

So that explains the Plumtree thing. Well, not entirely, because it has all sorts of other meanings, like everything else in *Ulysses*, but let's not worry about that just now. It is time for a brief account of the background of the book and then I'll tell you how I discovered it.

James Joyce (1882–1941) was an Irish writer who was born in Dublin but spent most of his creative life in self-imposed exile in places such as Paris, Trieste and Zürich. I would say that his chief subjects as a writer were the struggle to become an artist, human life as lived by ordinary people, the way it feels to be an outsider, and the million and one things you can do (or he could do) with the English language. His first books were relatively straightforward: poems (*Chamber Music*), short stories (*Dubliners*) and the autobiographical *A Portrait of the Artist as a Young Man*. With *Ulysses*, he took on something much more ambitious. He wanted to write a modern Irish epic comparable to the Greek poet Homer's long verse saga *The Odyssey*. This, of course, is the story of the Greek hero Odysseus, whose name in Latin is Ulysses. No problem so far, but when he presented his work, the publishers and critics and even some of his friends said, 'James, the language!' The writing in some of the chapters seemed very difficult at the time, when Modernism was still new, and it got more difficult as it went along. (The early chapters were serialised in the *Little Review*.) But worse than that, Jim's language was obscene! There was undue frankness about sexual matters (and other essential bodily functions), and the kind of words one may hear in the street but should not repeat in polite company were freely distributed in the text. This was very shocking in 1922 (decades before the *Lady Chatterley* trial), and with censorship and copies being seized by the police, *Ulysses* had a terrific struggle to get published. Eventually a brave lady called Sylvia Beach (of Shakespeare and Co) published the first edition in Paris. Daring English would cross the channel to get hold of a copy and smuggle it home through customs. Because those who managed to read the book had realised by now that Joyce equalled joy plus genius. *Ulysses* was finally published in America and the UK in the 1930s. And sometime in the 1940s, I suppose, my parents must have acquired a copy.

When I was about 14 or so, I used to open the glass-fronted doors of my parents' bookcase in the front room and have a browse. They had a small but varied collection of books including *The Business Encyclopaedia* (which my father must have thought would help him to get on in life), a set of Jewish prayer books (used once a year), a complete uniform edition of Dickens (special offer to readers of the *News Chronicle*) and a selection of hard-backed modern novels which my father brought home for my mother and himself to read. One day I pulled out a thick, dark green, hard-backed book and riffled through it idly. Almost at once, my eye was caught by some descriptions of sex from the female point of view. There were also some very naughty words which I'd never seen in print before. I continued browsing and found other passages which held my interest, despite being less arousing. Much of it seemed totally nonsensical, but the nonsense had an entertaining quality, so I kept on reading, just skipping about at random. Right at the beginning, three students, rather like my elder brothers, seemed to be having an amusing time living in a Martello tower (we had done those in history). One very long chapter was in the shape of a play set in a brothel (more titillation), with all sorts of bizarre scenes, some of them quite bewildering but very funny. What a strange book, I thought. Never come across anything like it before.

And then I turned a few more pages and found myself reading this:

Mr Leopold Bloom ate with relish the inner organs of beasts and fowls. He liked thick giblet soup, nutty gizzards, a stuffed roast heart, liver slices fried with crustcrumbs, fried hencod's roes. Most of all he liked grilled mutton kidneys which gave to his palate a fine tang of faintly scented urine.

Kidneys were on his mind as he moved about the kitchen softly, righting her breakfast things on the humpy tray. Gelid light and air were in the kitchen but out of doors gentle summer morning everywhere. Made him feel a bit peckish. The coals were reddening.

Another slice of bread and butter: three, four: right. She didn't like her plate full. Right. He turned from the tray, lifted the kettle off the hob and set it sideways on the fire. It sat there, dull and squat, its spout stuck out. Cup of tea soon. Good. Mouth dry. The cat walked stiffly round a leg of the table with tail on high.

– Mkgnao!

– O, there you are, Mr Bloom said, turning from the fire.

The cat mewed in answer and stalked again stiffly round a leg of the table, mewing. Prr. Scratch my head. Prr.

Mr Bloom watched curiously, kindly, the lithe black form. Clean to see: the gloss of her sleek hide, the white button under the butt of her tail, the green flashing eyes. He bent down to her, his hands on his knees.

– Milk for the pussens, he said.
– Mrkgnao! The cat cried.
  They call them stupid. They understand what we say better than we
understand them, She understands all she wants to. Vindictive too.
Wonder what I look like to her? Height of a tower? No, she can jump me.
– Afraid of the chickens she is, he said mockingly. Afraid of the
chookchooks. I never saw such a stupid pussens as the pussens.
  Cruel. Her nature. Curious mice never squeal. Seem to like it.
– Mrkrgnao! The cat said loudly.

That was my introduction to Mr Leopold Bloom, who was to become a life-long friend and companion. Mr Bloom is James Joyce's version of Odysseus (Ulysses). But instead of being a cunning, bloodthirsty hero he is a mild, inoffensive 38-year-old Dubliner. As we read on (and you will want to as well if you have stayed with me this far) we learn that he is Jewish (well partly), married to Molly (beautiful, adulterous, Irish, Jewish and Spanish) and not very successful either professionally or socially. He earns a rather precarious living working for the advertising department of a newspaper and is regarded by most of his acquaintances as a bit of a joke. Oh he's intelligent enough (a bit too full of information if you ask them) and quite harmless. But he never seems to be quite accepted as one of the lads. They whisper jokingly behind his back about his eccentric ways and his wife's affairs.

Nevertheless, Mr Bloom has a great deal going for him. He is intelligent, observant, compassionate and kind to animals (as we have seen). He has keen sensual appetites for food (in the frying pan) and for women (mainly in fantasy). He has a very rich inner life and, most important of all, he shares it with us, the readers of *Ulysses*. When I read the account of his day I feel I have been miniaturised, picked up and given a privileged seat in Bloom's mind. As he wanders about his kitchen or the streets of Dublin in 1904, I see everything from his point of view, hear all his thoughts, feel all his emotions. It is called 'the stream of consciousness' or 'the interior monologue' and it is just a wonderful ride. Mr Bloom was modelled partly on Joyce's father and he's a bit like my father and maybe yours too. Despite his modest position in life and his many weaknesses, he is the hero of the story and, as a result of Joyce's brilliant literary technique, the most accessible, most knowable hero in literature as well as one of the most loveable.

Now I'll tell you a little about how Mr Bloom spends his day and how we are going to spend it with him. After giving the cat some milk, he pops round to the pork butcher to get a nice kidney for his breakfast (threepence). Then he goes back and takes his wife Molly some tea in bed and they open their post. Bloom has a nice letter from their teenage daughter (Milly) and Molly has one from her lover, Hugh ('Blazes') Boylan, who will be visiting her in the afternoon for a spot of adultery. She pretends that he is coming only to show her the programme for a concert tour he is promoting her in (Molly is a fine singer), but Bloom knows exactly what's going on and it makes his heart heavy. However, he doesn't confront her. We learn later that Bloom and Molly have not made love since the death of their 11-day-old baby son, Rudy, 11 years ago.

After his breakfast (kidney only slightly burned) and a satisfying crap – yes we go everywhere with him, even into the outdoor loo where we read the newspaper while our physiology proceeds – Bloom sets off again to carry out various errands. And to make sure he is out of the house when Boylan calls to make love with Molly. As he walks through the Dublin streets, his thoughts are busy, fed by the sights and sounds, encounters with various acquaintances and his inner preoccupations. He calls at the post office to collect a letter. We learn that he is carrying out a clandestine flirtation by correspondence with a lady named Martha, who asks what perfume his wife uses and calls him 'naughty boy'. Unlike Molly's affair with Boylan, we feel sure that this one is going nowhere. His thoughts run on women, politics, music, science, the way things work, human nature, animals. He calls at a chemist to get some lotion made up for Molly and buys a cake of lemon-scented soap for fourpence. (Sweney's the chemist in Dublin still sells them in commemoration of this episode but now they will cost you rather more than fourpence.) Nothing sensational happens in Bloom's day but he is just enjoyable to be with, because he's basically a decent, nice little guy with a lot on his mind and a lively imagination which we are allowed to share completely.

Here he is meditating on childbirth and doctors as he walks down Westmoreland Street towards Trinity College:

Dth, dth, dth, dth! Three days imagine groaning on a bed with a vinegared handkerchief round her forehead, her belly swollen out! Phew! Dreadful simply! Child's head too big: forceps. Doubled up inside her trying to butt its way out blindly, groping for the way out. Kill me that would. Lucky Molly got over hers lightly. They ought to invent something to stop that. Life with hard labour. Twilight sleep idea: Queen Victoria was given that. Nine she had. Good layer ... Funny sight two of them together, their bellies out. Molly and Mrs Moisel. Mothers' meeting. Phthisis retires for the time being, then returns. How flat they look after all of a sudden! Peaceful eyes. Weight off their minds.... Snuffy Dr Murren. People knocking them up at all hours. For God'sake doctor. Wife in her throes. Then keep them waiting months for their fee. To attendance on your wife. No gratitude in people. Humane doctors, most of them. (Thanks, Leopold)

What else happens in Leopold's day? He attends a funeral with a group of 'friends' who clearly treat him as an outsider (although Martin Cunningham is always considerate). He tries to get a commission for an advertisement to be published in the *Freeman's Journal*, the paper which employs him. He has a modest lunch in Davy Byrne's pub. He meets an old flame, long married, and hears about another woman who is in the middle of a long and difficult labour. The men he meets continue to treat him at best with reserve and at worst with derision. They ask about Molly's concert tour in a way which hints that they know she's a good-looking, sexy woman whom Bloom can't possibly satisfy. On his way to the library he almost bumps into Blazes Boylan, the bounder, in his straw hat, tan shoes and turned-up trousers – and hastily avoids him. He buys a mildly pornographic novel for Molly at a street stall. At around four o'clock he has a meal in the Ormond Hotel and sees Boylan setting off for his tryst with Molly. He is distracted by listening to some impromptu singing. In another pub, he gets into an argument with the Citizen, a crazed Irish nationalist, and almost gets beaten up. He retreats to the strand (the Dublin bay beach) and enjoys a private erotic experience when a girl called Gerty MacDowell notices him watching her from a distance and accidentally-on-purpose shows him her knickers. At ten o'clock we find Bloom in the maternity hospital, enquiring about Mrs Purefoy's confinement and sitting round a table with a group of drunken medical students. These young men also include Stephen Dedalus, one of the other main characters in *Ulysses*. We meet Stephen in the first chapter, where he is sharing digs in the Martello tower. He is anxious to prove himself as a literary artist and represents the young James Joyce. (Stephen's early life is described in *A Portrait of the Artist as a Young Man*.) Unfortunately, Stephen seems to be drawn towards bad company and Bloom takes a paternal interest in him (especially as he has no son of his own). He follows Stephen to a bizarre brothel in order to keep an eye on him. However, inside the red light district (known as Nighttown) Bloom succumbs to an extraordinary series of dreams or hallucinations in which figures from his past mingle with strange sexual fantasies and delusions in which he experiences everything from world domination to total humiliation. (This chapter is also one of the funniest in a book which is brimming with humour of every kind.)

Finally, Bloom recovers his senses and extricates Stephen, who is on the point of being arrested after a quarrel with two soldiers, one of whom has knocked him down. They retire to Bloom's house for a cup of cocoa and a meeting of minds. Bloom would clearly like to adopt the troubled Stephen and invites him to stay the night: but Stephen declines. It is now about 2 am and Bloom reviews the events of the day as he retires to the marital bedroom. He caresses Molly's bottom: she wakes and they have a brief conversation before he settles down to sleep, lying beside her but upside down in the bed with his head beside her feet. 'Womb? Weary? He rests. He has travelled.'

The last chapter belongs to Molly. In a long and wondrous monologue with hardly any punctuation she meditates on her life and loves and decides that Bloom is probably the best of the bunch, despite his faults and his partial erectile dysfunction (or whatever it is). The book closes with a touching account of the young Bloom and Molly lying in each other's arms on Howth Head; of his proposal and her eager acceptance:

I thought as well him as another and then I asked him with my eyes to ask again yes and then he asked me would I yes to say yes my mountain flower and first I put my arms around him yes and drew him down to me so he could feel my breasts all perfume yes and his heart was going like mad and yes I said yes I will Yes.

I always feel a bit giddy after reading that and have to lie down for a while. But what, you may be asking, has this all got to do with Homer's Odyssey?

Ulysses and *The Odyssey*

Homer's story, you may remember, tells the tale of how Odysseus (Ulysses) took a terrible long time getting home from the Trojan wars on account of adverse weather conditions, unusual traffic flow problems in the Mediterranean and unforeseen interventions by Greek gods. Meanwhile, back home in Ithaca, his wife, Penelope, fended off hundreds of eager suitors and his son, Telemachus, set off on a quest to find out what had happened to his old man.

You might have noticed that there is a loose correspondence here between Joyce's cast and Homer's. Bloom is the wanderer, detained by various adventures (in his case in Dublin), Stephen the son in search of a father and Molly the wife who is undoubtedly entertaining suitors but welcomes her husband home at the end of the day. When he was writing *Ulysses*, Joyce built in lots of other references and correspondences, some easier to find than others. He even produced a 'schema' or key to the structure of the book, in which each chapter had the title of one of the episodes in *The Odyssey*, and lent it to a friend who was going to give a lecture on the book before it was generally available. So the funeral chapter (six of 18) is called, appropriately, 'Hades'; the 12th chapter, which deals with Bloom's encounter with the aggressive 'Citizen' in Barney Kearnan's pub is called 'Cyclops', after the one-eyed giant who imprisons Odysseus and his companions in a cave and devours several of them before they escape. And the final chapter, Molly's solo, is of course 'Penelope'. The schema contains other bits of information too, like how each chapter has its own art, colour, symbol and organ of the body.

But when *Ulysses* was finally published, blow me if Joyce didn't remove all the chapter headings, so you won't find them in your copy. All you get is a division into three sections headed by Roman numerals. Rather frustrating, because the chapter titles are very helpful in navigating about the book and jolly useful for Joyce enthusiasts to use when discussing their favourite topic. However, you will almost certainly find the schema reprinted in the introduction to your *Ulysses* and – I tell you this in confidence – what most of us do is write in the chapter headings in pencil. I suggest you do the same, because I'm going to use them from now on. In fact you don't need to know anything about Homer to enjoy *Ulysses*, but it certainly adds an extra dimension if you are aware of the parallels.

The other hero

Yes, there is another hero, ever-present in the pages of *Ulysses* and that is the English language. With Joyce's expert guidance, English puts on a brilliant performance the like of which you have never seen. The language speaks in a hundred different voices, appears in many different disguises, has numerous adventures and performs acrobatic feats of astonishing virtuosity. Or, to put it another way, Joyce was in love with the language and wanted to use it in every way he could think of. I have already described the wonderfully effective use of Bloom's inner thoughts and this is the main narrative technique in several chapters, with frequent appearances in others. But the language speaks with all sorts of other voices as well. For a start, some of the other characters, mainly Stephen and Molly; tell you their thoughts directly as well: Stephen, troubled and intellectual; Molly, amorous and dreamy. But other, unnamed narrators intrude all over the place. Some sound like ordinary citizens of Dublin, others seem very bookish and serious. Some passages are hilarious parodies of all kinds of inflated and pompous purple prose. The 'Nausicaa' chapter (Bloom's erotic experience on the seashore) is written in a sort of parody of 'women's magazine' romantic fiction. The 'Circe' (brothel) chapter is almost entirely in the form of a surreal play. The 'Sirens' chapter, which has a lot of singing in it, was written by Joyce as if he was composing music and is full of beautiful sounds, rhythms and musical devices. And the maternity hospital episode ('Oxen of the Sun' – strange name, I know, you'll have to look it up) is a spectacular display of literary impersonation which imitates just about every style of written English from Chaucer to the twentieth century, before disintegrating altogether.

How to read *Ulysses*

OK, I know what you are thinking. No wonder the book has such an awesome reputation for being difficult to read if the language mutates into something different every time you turn the page. And you have to write in the chapter titles yourself. And the titles all come from a different book anyway. Can I possibly read this book through without getting lost?

Here is my suggestion for first-timers. Don't try to swallow it all at once. Bite off a few tasty chunks to start with. Read Chapter 1 (we can number them from 1 to 18), which starts with Stephen's medical student friend 'stately, plump Buck Mulligan' emerging from the Martello tower on the Dublin seashore for a shave. He teases poor Stephen about his artistic aspirations and reproaches him for refusing to kneel and pray for his dying mother at her request. This leads naturally to Chapter 2 ('Nestor'), in which Stephen teaches school and has a dysfunctional conversation with Mr Deasy, a rather repellent headmaster. Skip Chapter 3 (unless you know a lot about Aristotle) and go straight on to 4 and 5, the first two Bloom chapters, both delightful and easy to read. Chapter 6 ('Hades') is the funeral (you'll enjoy that).

Then you can just browse along, hanging on to Bloom whenever he appears and skipping quickly through the newspaper office ('Aeolus', Chapter 7) and the Shakespearean discussion in the National Library ('Scylla and Charybdis', Chapter 9) if you find it hard to follow. But do feel free, especially in the difficult chapters, to linger over a paragraph that catches your eye and takes your fancy. Savour it and move on to the next. Listen to the music of the 'Sirens' (Chapter 11) and enjoy the company of the bronze- and gold-haired barmaids. Watch out for Blazes Boylan making a disturbing appearance. Join Bloom for the argument in the pub ('Cyclops', Chapter 12), but note that the narration is now given by an anonymous drinker whose account is interspersed with all sorts of entertaining parodies. For instance, Joyce interrupts the narrative to give a description of the terrible old bigoted nationalist, which seems to come straight from some sort of bizarre Irish folk epic: 'The figure seated on a large boulder at the foot of a round tower was that of a broadshouldered deepchested stronglimbed frankeyed redhaired freely freckled shaggybearded wisemouthed largenosed longheaded deepvoiced barekneed brawnyhanded ruddy faced sinewyarmed hero ...', etc.

Go on to Bloom's seaside dalliance with Gerty McDowell (Chapter 13, *Woman's Weekly*-style, easy to read). Read a few paragraphs of Chapter 14 ('Oxen of the Sun'), in which you'll meet some obscene and noisy medical students but if you find some of the prose styles hard-going, hurry on and don't get bogged down. Chapter 15 (Circe's brothel dramatised) is completely different, full of hallucinations, brilliantly written and very entertaining. Here is Bloom's barrister defending him against a charge of gross indecency:

My client is an infant, a poor foreign immigrant who started scratch as a stowaway and is now trying to turn an honest penny. The trumped up misdemeanor was due to a momentary aberration of heredity brought on by hallucination ... There have been cases of shipwreck and somnambulism in my client's family ... He himself, my lord, is a physical wreck from cobbler's weak chest. His submission is that he is of Mongolian extraction and irresponsible for his actions. Not all there in fact.

It reads uncannily like one of the letters I write for my patients when they have to appear in court.

Now you have three chapters to go. You can hurry through the first one ('Eumaeus'), in which Bloom and Stephen sojourn in a cabman's shelter; but spend time with the second ('Ithaca'), in which everything is in question-and-answer form with the answers minutely detailed. Joyce said it was his favourite chapter and it is one of mine too. Do you like lists? Then this one is for you. The last chapter ('Penelope') is, of course, Molly Bloom's drowsy meditation as she lies alongside her upside-down sleeping husband. You can browse through it just before *you* go to sleep. You won't take it all in because you are so drowsy yourself, but that doesn't matter. You have had your first odyssey through *Ulysses* and you have become a member of the club. From now on you can pick the book up any time you like and read a chapter here or there as the mood takes you. You can hug yourself and chuckle over the jokes and puns as you uncover more and more of them. Eventually, you might even read the more difficult chapters, maybe in more detail than I ever have. You might also be interested to read one of the many commentaries on the book written by other members of the club. I hope that for you, as for them (and for me), reading *Ulysses* will become one of life's very special pleasures.

About the author

James Joyce was born in Dublin and educated at Jesuit schools and University College Dublin. His father was a talented man but he drank too much. He tried a number of different professions without much success and the Joyces were constantly having to move house. James went to Paris in 1902 intending to study medicine, but wisely decided to be a writer instead. He returned to Dublin for his mother's funeral and stayed briefly in the Martello tower (see *Ulysses*, Chapter 1) with Oliver St John Gogarty, a medical student friend who was the model for Buck Mulligan. Shortly afterwards he met his life-long love, Nora Barnacle, and the pair left Ireland more or less for good, although he carried Dublin around with him in his head. James and Nora (who never read any of his books) lived in Trieste, Zürich and finally Paris, and they had two children. His first books were a volume of poems (*Chamber Music*, 1907) and then a collection of short stories (*Dubliners*, 1914). These were followed by the semi-autobiographical *A Portrait of the Artist as a Young Man*, which introduces the character of Stephen Dedalus and contained the famous hellfire sermon. He then got down to serious work on *Ulysses*, whose stormy reception and difficult publication I have described above. Joyce's final work, *Finnegan's Wake,* took many years to complete and was finally published in 1939. In this revolutionary book the English language seems to dissolve and flow like water. It is very perplexing to read and the 'plot' is hard to follow, but it is full of beautiful sounds, outrageous puns and hilarious jokes. In later life, Joyce suffered badly from glaucoma and became more or less blind. He died in Zürich from a perforated duodenal ulcer. Although *Ulysses* was originally banned in Ireland, Joyce is now a national literary treasure and you can celebrate 'Bloomsday' in Dublin every year on 16 June.

The text

Ulysses by James Joyce was first published in 1922 but that edition contained numerous errors. Joyce spent a lot of time correcting it from his own drafts. A 'corrected' text was published by Penguin in 1986. It is easy to read and handle, and contains a good introduction (with schema) by Declan Kiberd. Alternatively, Oxford World Classics have published a reproduction of the 1922 text, which points out significant errors and has the most comprehensive notes.

Further reading

Homer *The Odyssey.* Translation by Robert Fagles (1996). Penguin, Harmondsworth.

Ellman R (1959) *James Joyce.* Oxford University Press, Oxford (revised 1982). A classic and excellent biography.

8

Indian Camp

by Ernest Hemingway

Brian Glasser

I propose in this piece to come at things from a slightly different angle – that of a communication skills tutor who uses literature in small-group undergraduate medical school (and, on occasion, GP registrar) teaching. Having described the way a session might work, I offer some broader reflections about the role of literature in medical education, via a discussion of Ernest Hemingway's *Indian Camp*.

Starting points

Medical students in the UK have typically had to forego formal study of the arts at the relatively tender age of 16, when A-level subjects are selected and sciences are deemed to be of paramount importance. This is not to say that they do not retain an interest in (and talent for) matters artistic, as anyone who has attended a student art exhibition or concert performance or end-of-year show can testify. But because of the hiatus in their considerations of Literature with a capital L, they approach it with some trepidation.

Their anxiety is often cloaked in the question, usually asked rhetorically, 'But what does this have to do with studying medicine?' To placate them, I choose a text which is overtly relevant in subject matter, and accessible in size and style.

A short story by Ernest Hemingway entitled *Indian Camp*, fits the bill nicely. At around 1500 words (five pages in my budget-price paperback edition of selected stories by the author[1]), it can be read in a few minutes. Hemingway's prose is straightforward enough, at least in terms of syntax and vocabulary – so nothing there to deter the apprehensive first-time reader. And the story-line could have been custom-made by a medical educational board: in the Michigan countryside, a doctor takes his brother and his son Nick to watch him deliver a (Native American) Indian woman's baby in her shanty home. He has to perform a Caesarean with improvised equipment; the mother and child both survive; the Indian father, bedridden in a bunk above his wife because of an injury, commits suicide, an event which goes unnoticed until the delivery is over. The doctor and his son go home.

Ways in

Most of us know the unease that accompanies our first encounter with a work of art of reputation – will we 'understand' it, or will we instead reveal our stupidity by missing the point entirely? People sometimes believe that to make sense of a text you need to learn about the author's life (Hemingway's father was a doctor who would sometimes take the young Ernest on visits with him; and who, like Hemingway himself, committed suicide); or about his other work (the story is part of a carefully structured collection of short stories called *In Our Time*); or about his place in the literary pantheon (there are journals devoted solely to Hemingway studies); or be well-versed in literary theory (are you a New Critic or Structuralist, a Feminist or Formalist?). Certainly, finding out about these things can affect one's response to a piece of writing; but ultimately, they are probably no more or less relevant than the resonances the story has with things from one's own history.

At any rate, medical students can be forgiven for feeling this unease acutely, because of the aforementioned lack of arts education during their late teens and beyond. But like most things, feeling confident about reading literature comes with a little guidance, and lots of practice in the shape of grappling with examples. The tutor's job is to compensate for medical students' lack of the latter with some careful attention to the former.

The first and by far the most important piece of advice is to read the text closely for it is, to put it in the scientific idiom, the primary source of data. So with a minimal introduction to the session, I tell the students to read through the story once. Because it has a powerful emotional impact – the suicide is shocking in both senses of the word – I then ask them to tell me, in one or two words, what it made them feel. Responses usually include 'sad', 'upset', 'surprised' and, interestingly, 'angry'. I also ask them, as a group, to outline the events that take place in the story, so that we can iron out any misunderstandings and agree on a common base for discussion. Now we have our two key ingredients for the session: the story itself, and people's response to it.

The next task is to get them to work out what made them respond as they did – to identify the connections between our ingredients. Quickly, they plunge back into the text, but this time reading it in subgroups, each pair or trio with a specific focus. The themes I usually get them to reflect on include: what is there in the story about cultural relations between the whites and the Indians? Chart the psychological state of Nick and his father, and dynamics of their interaction. How is medicine characterised via the doctor's persona? I stress that students must provide specific instances in the text to support their assertions.

This is the part of the session where you can hear the brains whirring and the discussion becoming animated – first in the subgroups and then during the feedback to the full group. Worries about 'not understanding' the text have been replaced by strongly held opinions! The tutor becomes a presiding magistrate, whose task is to ensure that every voice is heard and all admissible evidence is elicited. I also get the students to think about how Hemingway uses language to achieve the results they are describing. Summing up these last issues – or getting the students to – is a useful way of bringing this part of the session to a close.

Depending on time constraints, I sometimes give the students a page to read from a *BMJ* paper (to draw attention to the language doctors employ with one another) and/or a page from Jane Austen (for its psychological revelations). The contrast in the use of language puts the Hemingway in sharp relief, and reinforces many of the points about writing style that have arisen during earlier discussion. The seminar usually ends with students in enthusiastic mood, having had an agreeable and enlightening time, their initial suspicions forgotten. From an educationalist's point of view, one can be reasonably confident that they have assimilated the story and reflected on its implications for them as future doctors.

Sifting the treasure of *Indian Camp*

To give a fuller idea of what the students have to work with, I'll now take a closer look at *Indian Camp*.

The first thing that strikes most readers of the story is the author's style, which is not the sort that people associate with 'serious art'. He begins in the manner in which he means to continue:

> *At the lake shore there was another rowboat drawn up. The two Indians stood waiting.*
>
> *Nick and his father got in the stern of the boat and the Indians shoved it off and one of them got in to row. Uncle George sat in the stern of the camp rowboat. The young Indian shoved the camp boat off and got in to row Uncle George.*

Length is often equated with complexity with regard to language – for instance, when reading scores are used to assess patient information leaflets. On this basis, Hemingway could have had a glorious career with the Health Education Authority. The paragraphs are short. The sentences are short. The words that make them up are short, and repetitive in a way which breaks the rules a schoolchild learns about essay writing. Crucially, the sentences have no subordinate clauses, whose usual function is to provide comment of some sort about the main clauses (as in this sentence!). If a sentence is longer, it is only because Hemingway has strung together main clauses, separating them with 'and'. This device emphasises the 'levelling out' of the text that Hemingway seems to be striving for.

And yet despite this apparently flat, charmless writing the reader is not unengaged. This is partly because the rhythm of the prose commands attention; and also because witholding information from the reader forces us to concentrate hard on the text to make gradual sense of it. In the first sentence, the word 'another' is slightly unsettling – for it implies we know something which in fact we have not been told (i.e. what is the original boat that is being referred to?). We are given no date, time, place, background information on the protagonists, or explanation of why this journey is being undertaken – the sorts of things that one would usually include if telling a story. Nor are we provided with any further biographical information about these (or any other) characters in the rest of the story.

If we initially are struck by how little information there appears to be in these opening paragraphs, they nevertheless tell us more than we first realise. For example, we can deduce that Nick's perspective is probably going to be at the centre of the story, since he is the first person to be named and because other characters are named in relation to him (notably his father and Uncle George). We also glean from the latter's appellations that Nick is probably a child. The Indians, by contrast, are designated only by their race, although one is distinguished by his relative youth – perhaps as a parallel to Nick. We notice that the Indians are – by tacit agreement – subservient, waiting for the whites to arrive and then negotiating the embarkation and rowing unaided, even though one of the boats belongs to the whites. Of course the style of the writing, too, tells us something about what we are letting ourselves in for if we continue reading this story: a mood, an attitude perhaps, with we know not what implications yet.

This is the style that Hemingway is famous for 'inventing'. If it seems familiar it is because it spawned the American 'hard-boiled' school of detective stories that have so defined the modern thriller. The fundamental strategy is to eliminate what semiotic critics call 'discourse', as opposed to 'story'. Essentially, this means that Hemingway confines himself to describing the physical setting and the events that take place within it, while eschewing all exploration of the psychological activity of the protagonists. There are only two occasions in the story when Hemingway relaxes his policy a little to allow a glimpse of emotion. The second is at the end of the story, when Nick has an (understated) reaction to all that has gone before. But the first is when the doctor has finished what has been a long and harrowing Caesarean:

> *He was feeling exalted and talkative as football players are in the dressing-room after a game.*
> *'That's one for the medical journal, George' he said. 'Doing a Caesarean with a jack-knife and sewing it up with nine-foot, tapered gut leaders.'*

It's hardly purple prose, but 'exalted' and 'talkative' are the most upbeat words in the story, and the use of a simile seems positively cavalier in the context of Hemingway's bone-dry style. But what happens next appears to be retribution for allowing such unguarded pride to express itself, however briefly:

> *Uncle George was standing against the wall, looking at his arm [which had earlier been bitten by the pregnant woman during her labour pains].*
> *'Oh, you're a great man, alright,' he said.*
> *'Ought to have a look at the proud father. They're usually the worst sufferers in these little affairs,' the doctor said. 'I must say he took it all pretty quietly.'*
> *He pulled back the blanket from the Indian's head. His hand came away wet. He mounted the edge of the lower bunk with the lamp in one hand and looked in. The Indian lay with his face to the wall. His throat had been cut from ear to ear. The blood had flowed down into a pool where his body sagged the bunk. His head rested on his left arm. The open razor lay, edge up, in the blankets.*

Suddenly we realise the price of failing to pay any attention to the Indian father during the 'little affair'. We the readers have become unavoidably implicated in this terrible oversight, too; the shock is as great for us as the protagonists in the story. Hemingway had mentioned the father twice earlier, but with only the smallest of details, which appeared entirely insignificant at the time. A second reading shows he had chosen those details carefully, and we berate ourselves for only registering their importance in retrospect.

So we discover that the purpose of the stylistic restraint in the story goes beyond the desire to prevent complacency on the part of the reader. It has served to set up the blow to the emotional solar plexus that the author had planned. Even now, Hemingway supplies no discussion of the reasons for the man's suicide, or the responses to its discovery by others. The text continues:

'Take Nick out of the shanty, George,' the doctor said.

There was no need of that. Nick, standing in the door of the kitchen, had a good view of the upper bunk when his father, the lamp in one hand, tipped the Indian's head back.

It was beginning to be daylight when they walked along the logging road back to the lake.

A little later on, Nick asks:

'Why did he kill himself, Daddy?'

'I don't know, Nick. He couldn't stand things, I guess.'

'Do many men kill themselves, Daddy?'

'Not very many, Nick.'

'Is dying hard, Daddy?'

'No, I think it's pretty easy, Nick. It all depends.'

And the story concludes:

In the early morning on the lake sitting in the stern of the boat with his father rowing, he felt quite sure that he would never die.

It is evident that Hemingway is the master of the domain of the unspoken. Reading becomes very uncomfortable, as we are denied any vicarious emotional outlet. Hemingway's own comments on the art of writing are illuminating here:

If you leave out important things or events that you know about, the story is strengthened. If you leave or skip something because you do not know it, the story will be worthless. The test of any story is how very good the stuff that you, not your editors, omit.[2]

Hemingway is dealing with highly emotive issues, and there is a huge discrepancy between the complexity of the subject matter and the simplicity of the language used to convey it. The centrality of this discrepancy leads us back to our starting point.

Literature and medical students

Indian Camp is relevant for medical students studying communication skills on (at least!) three different levels. First, and most obviously, the story tells us of the potential benefits and dangers of what we can loosely refer to as the medical model. For instance, the doctor in the story performs surgery which is little short of heroic. He has probably saved two lives, and yet asks for and expects no thanks or recompense, beyond the respect of his peers via a journal publication. This is the selfless stuff that medical myth is made of. He is understandably exhilarated by his own accomplishment, and who could deny him this? Yet the talk of football players is a warning to the reader. It traces the doctor's 'buzz' back to an immature psychological source, his achievement being akin to a sporting success. This might not matter too much, except for the tragic event that is unfolding alongside the medical action. For in this story, the football mentality saves two lives, but contributes to the loss of one, and the enormous damage inflicted on several others (the Indian woman and her new child, who lose their partner/father; the Indian community as a whole; and Nick, who witnesses the gory discovery). As mentioned, Hemingway never explains why the Indian commits suicide, but we are given several clues in the text which suggest that (putting it simply) his manhood has been intolerably compromised.

Writing 70 years before *Changing Childbirth* was published, Hemingway is alert to the insensitivity of the doctor's conduct to the mother, to whom he doesn't say a word. At one point the woman cries out in pain:

'Oh Daddy, can't you give her something to make her stop screaming?' asked Nick.

'No. I haven't any anaesthetic,' his father said. 'But her screams are not important. I don't hear them because they are not important.'

In this exchange, he encapsulates the ethos of medical detachment, which doctors are taught to cultivate now as then. It is an ethos which can be justified for two sound reasons: first, to ensure that a doctor's judgement and technique are not impaired by personal considerations; and second – though inexplicitly – because it affords the doctor some emotional protection from the suffering that constantly surrounds him. Yet we have begun to see the paradox of adopting this attitude. We recognise the personal strain that can follow in the wake of detachment, and there is concern nowadays about the high levels of stress-related problems within the medical profession. Parallel to this, patients frequently complain about doctors being uncaring to the point of seeming callous. Strength can beget weakness.

This issue – that of the inadequacy of the medical model – is embodied in the correlation between denial of emotion in Hemingway's prose style and in the doctor's personal style. There is a terrible tension between the surface activity and the way it is being described, and the psychological realities underneath – a case study in the axiom that 'there's more to this than meets the eye'.

We could perhaps teach this lesson by getting students to read a large number of patient notes. But Hemingway, in his role as artist, has done all the work for us and laid it out as neatly as in a textbook.

Unlike Hemingway, I am too weak-willed to deny myself the titillation of a biographical observation. For the fascinating irony is he lived his life determinedly as a man's man – womanising, drinking, big-game hunting and the like, vaunting those who did their job professionally, whether they were bullfighters or fishermen, and scorning weakness. But he went through marriages like mince pies, suffered from depression and eventually succumbed to the strain of keeping up with his own reputation. In other words, he lived out the very dichotomy he describes in this story.

The second level on which *Indian Camp* is useful is that it offers an opportunity for students to think about narratives. We all make sense of the world by shaping our random experience into stories. They have a beginning, a middle and sometimes, though not always, an end. If we fall sick, we try to answer the questions

'Why me, why now?'; and we have notions about what might help us recover. When we cannot find answers to these questions, we may visit the doctor. In training for history taking at the Royal Free Hospital, we discuss with students how patients often bring partial explanations of their illness to the doctor and are in search of information in order to complete their story.

In some proximity to this second level lies the third. Good artists (in any medium) are, by definition, good communicators, and consequently tell stories well. By breaking down the whole into some of its parts, students begin to see how much is going on in the text and how carefully assembled the whole is. This increased awareness of the craft of writing serves to demystify it somewhat and to make it feel less alien to students, while at the same time making them better appreciate the scale of the author's achievement. Students become sensitised to the effect of words when used in particular ways. Thus in studying the nuts and bolts of how a master tells a story, they can better understand everyday storytelling and, by extension, be more aware of the impact that communication issues have on patients and doctors.

As I hope I have conveyed, *Indian Camp* is a wonderfully rich piece of work that repays close consideration. It is 'about' many things, many of them out of the range of both a single teaching session and this paper. But I hope I've persuaded you that literature is an invaluable tool for medical student teaching, and that this particular slice of it is well worth a read for the rest of us.

About the author

Ernest Hemingway (1899–1961) was born in a Chicago suburb, and his father was a doctor. He began writing as a cub reporter for the *Kansas City Star* in 1917 and then, the following year, he volunteered to be an ambulance driver on the Italian front. He was badly wounded and twice decorated for his services. He later reported on the Greek–Turkish war (1922) before settling in Paris, where he devoted himself to writing novels and perfecting his characteristic macho prose style. He was friendly with Gertrude Stein and Ezra Pound, who both gave him encouragement. His spare-time interests were bullfighting, deep-sea fishing and big-game hunting, and all these activities appear in his books. His best books are *A Farewell to Arms, For Whom the Bell Tolls* (which draws on experiences in Spain during the Civil War) and *The Old Man and the Sea*. He was awarded the Nobel Prize for literature in 1954.

References

1   Hemingway E (1924) Indian Camp. In *The First Fortynine Stories by Ernest Hemingway* (1944) Jonathan Cape, London. Extracts reprinted by kind permission of The Random House Group Ltd.

2   Hemingway E (1959) *The Art of the Short Story.* First published in *Paris Review.* **79** (1981).

9

The Brothers Karamazov

by Fyodor Dostoyevsky

About the author

Fyodor Dostoyevsky is, of course, one of the great Russian writers of the nineteenth century, and it is time for us to make his acquaintance. He was born in Moscow in 1821, the second son of a poor, struggling doctor. (The close connections between medicine and literature never cease to amaze and delight me.) Young Fyodor (in English his name would be Theodore) qualified as a military engineer but soon decided that he would rather be a writer. He had an early success (*Poor Folk*, 1846) but then in 1849 got himself arrested for belonging to a group of political dissidents. Along with five comrades, he was sentenced to death by firing squad. Then, just as they were about to be shot, they were all told that they had been reprieved by Tsar Nicholas I and Fyodor was taken off to Omsk for four years of penal servitude. He was transported on a sledge, his legs in iron fetters, in temperatures which went down to $-40°F$. About this time, he started to get generalised convulsive epilepsy (described in *The Idiot*). When he was released from prison and was able to take his leg irons off, he soon became a writer again. In 1865, he began work on *Crime and Punishment* (the one we all read as students, wondering if we could ever behave like Raskolnikov). Dostoyevsky's personal life wasn't as grim as his hero's but it was fairly bad. He was still having frequent fits, his first marriage was a disaster and he was in chronic debt. Then, in 1866, when he was struggling to write a new novel to meet a deadline, his friends sent him a typist, a 20-year-old girl called Anna. They fell in love and Anna tried her best to get Fyodor's life into some sort of order, but unfortunately, he developed a taste for gambling (that book she was typing was called *The Gambler*).They travelled all over Western Europe and he went through thousands of roubles, as well as writing some brilliant books (mainly at night). At last they decided to go back to Russia and, after a final fling at the Wiesbaden casino (in which he lost the money for their train fare), they eventually did go home. And he really did give up gambling. The rest of their married life seems to have been very happy. They had great times in bed; he had an erotic obsession with her feet, but apparently she didn't mind. (I wish I had time to tell you more about things like that.) In 1878, Fyodor started writing his last and greatest book: *The Brothers Karamazov*. Like so many great nineteenth-century novels this was serialised in a magazine and copies were soon in great demand. Dostoyevsky had become a famous and respected writer, although his religious fervour and his eccentric political views confused people (he believed in the Russian People but not in parliamentary government). He died, probably of pulmonary tuberculosis, in 1881, and 20 000 people are said to have followed his funeral procession. After his death his reputation went up and down. Stalin thought he was brilliant but dangerous and had him banned. But, after the death of the considerably more dangerous dictator, Dostoyevsky was restored to his position as one of Russia's best-loved and most-read novelists.

The Brothers Karamazov

I have chosen this one to share with you because it is my favourite of all Dostoyevsky's books. It is another big one, as big as *Ulysses*, but it is excellent value and satisfies all sorts of literary desires. Think of it as a kind of giant gift hamper packed with all sorts of different tasty treats. Within the book's 900 or so pages Dostoyevsky has provided a gripping family saga about three tempestuous brothers, the anatomy of a small Russian town, a murder mystery, a courtroom drama and some passionate arguments about the nature of God. As if that's not enough, you also get the astonishing Legend of the Grand Inquisitor, which will make your hair stand on end, I promise you. I couldn't honestly say there's a proper love story – you have to go to Tolstoy for that – but there's plenty of sex, violence and religion; not to mention strange peasants, mad monks, children and a dog. Most of the time everyone is in a state of high excitement bordering on frenzy. But the passages about the Father Zossima, which paint a portrait of a genuinely wise and good man, provide some refreshing interludes of calm. Everything is held together by an anonymous storyteller who obviously lives in the little town where the story takes place. He has a wry sense of humour and is an excellent guide to have at your elbow.

I am not going to go through the whole story chapter by chapter, but I shall provide some readers' notes on each of the main characters and themes. So come with me and let's meet those legendary Karamazov boys and their terrible old father.

The three brothers and their father

Karamazov senior is an unattractive old man. I say 'old man', but in fact he is only about 57, two years younger than I am now. He is a shady business man and property dealer whom Dostoyevsky describes as 'worthless and depraved'. There is a description of his repulsive appearance, which I won't quote in full, but it includes 'a long, cruel and sensual mouth with full lips, between which could be seen stumps of black and almost decayed teeth'. However, he does have a clownish sense of humour and an ability to puncture pomposity. Old Karamazov has been married twice, but by the time our story opens his first wife has run off with someone else, his second has been dead for many years and he is currently lusting after a young beauty called Grushenka (of whom much more later.)

All three of his sons (one from the first marriage, two from the second) were brought up at first by his old manservant Grigory and later by distant relatives. The boys are called Dmitri, Ivan and Alexander.

Dmitri (known as Mitya) is the eldest. When we first meet him, he is an ex-army officer of 27. He has just come back to 'our little town' in the hope of persuading his miserly father to part with a large sum of money which he believes is his inheritance. Mitya is the wildest of the three boys; impulsive, passionate, reckless in pursuit of young women (who find him very attractive) and, like his creator, always strapped for cash. He can also be quite violent; he is very angry with his father and it is not surprising that he is suspect number one when old Karamazov is murdered (yes, that's the murder story, coming up). I suppose if he was a patient you would probably think of Mitya as someone with a psychopathic personality disorder and be very wary of him. Probably you would seriously consider striking him, and maybe his whole family, off your list and I wouldn't blame you. Nothing but trouble, the lot of them. But I have a soft spot for Mitya, all the same, because in his own way he is completely open and honest and he can be quite generous.

The second brother, Ivan, is four years younger than Mitya and he is the intellectual of the family. He has been away at university and seems to be doing quite well as a freelance journalist. Some of his articles have attracted attention in literary circles. Ivan appears to be rather cold and emotionally distant, with nothing like the warmth and impulsiveness of his elder brother. However, he is very fond of the youngest brother (Alexander, known as Alyosha), with whom he has a famous discussion on religion (I say discussion, but Ivan does nearly all the talking; Alyosha just listens and tries to hang on to his faith).

What about Alyosha? He is only 20 when the story begins. He is quite different from the other two and is a really nice boy, even if he is a bit pious. As the youngest of three brothers myself, I tend to identify a bit with Alyosha, but I don't claim to be as saintly as he is. Alyosha's mother died when he was four, but he always remembers her face. He is very shy and quiet, likes reading and as a schoolboy used to get very upset if anyone talked about sex. When we are introduced to him he is wearing a cassock and living in the local monastery, where the revered Father Zossima is his mentor. However, he is not going to be a monk for ever and the good Father is always telling him that he must 'go out into the world'. Alyosha's job is to be the family peacemaker: he listens to everyone and condemns nobody. But he's not at all priggish and I'm sure you are going to like him. In fact, you will probably be disappointed to find that Alyosha plays only a small part in the second half of the novel. This is because Dostoyevsky planned to write a sequel which was to be all about What Alyosha Did Next, – but unhappily he did not live to produce it.

The girlfriends

I'll tell you about the young ladies next, because they play a crucial role in the development of the plot. The main problem is that Mitya is involved in relationships with two girls, Katerina and Grushenka. Katerina is tall and aristocratic, the daughter of a lieutenant-colonel. When her father badly needs 4500 roubles (which he has 'borrowed' from the regimental funds and cannot repay), Mitya lets it be known that he will supply the money if Katerina will come to him to collect it in person. She humbles herself to do so for her father's sake and kneels at Mitya's feet in gratitude. This is so moving for both of them that they fall in love and get engaged. Poor old Ivan, the intellectual falls for Katerina as well, but he has no chance. Then Mitya encounters the 22-year-old Grushenka, a local beauty who also has some sort of liaison with his father, old Fyodor Karamazov. Grushenka's beauty is much more sensual and Mitya finds her irresistible: 'the body of that hell-cat woman is nothing but curves from top to bottom, right down to the little toe on her left foot. I saw that toe and I kissed it, but that's all, I swear', he confesses to Alyosha. (You remember what I said about Dostoyevsky and women's feet.) So Mitya finds himself with commitments to both women and an angry rivalry with his father over Grushenka. This anger leads Mitya to make death threats against his father, so it's little wonder that he is suspect number one when the old man is found murdered. What about Alyosha? Does he have a girlfriend? Yes, he does. She is a young girl called Lise, who is very keen to be betrothed to him, although her mother thinks that at 14 she is much too young, and one can't help agreeing. When we first meet her, Lise is in a wheelchair and she appears to be recovering from an attack of polio. Happily she seems to get back on her feet again quite soon. Lise is very lively and endearing and tends to tease Alyosha about his cassock. It would be nice to know what happened to the young lovers, but I'm afraid their story was never finished.

The plot: murder most foul

Now that I've introduced you to the main characters I think it's time for me to give you a brief outline of the main plot, which is about the violent death of old Fyodor Karamazov. One night, he is waiting in his house with mounting excitement because he believes that Grushenka might be about to respond to his invitation to pay him a visit. Underneath his pillow he has an envelope containing 3000 roubles (in rainbow-coloured 100 rouble notes). The envelope is marked 'to my angel Grushenka if she will come to me'. But the person who comes that night is the murderer, who bashes the old man's head in and makes off with the money. Was it Mitya? It looks very much like it because he was certainly lurking round the house hoping to intercept Grushenka if she should decide to visit his father. Not only lurking but carrying a large brass pestle. We stay with Mitya right up to the point where he stands, holding the blunt instrument and gazes balefully through the window at the figure of the old man, his father. Then Dostoyevsky teases us by making a jump cut to Mitya rushing away, without showing us whether or not he actually commits the murder.

In his flight, Mitya is confronted by his father's old servant Grigory, who tries to restrain him. He uses the pestle to club poor Grigory on the head (fortunately not fatally) and then runs off. He is seen about town by various people, covered in blood, in a state of wild agitation and with a wad of rainbow-coloured notes, which he is spending freely. He takes off to a village in the country in pursuit of Grushenka. At the local inn they have a wild party which lasts several days and only ends when the police arrive to arrest Mitya on the charge of murdering his father. An investigation and a big trial are to follow, all described in loving detail by the master storyteller. But is Mitya really guilty? For there is another suspect, the epileptic servant Smerdyakov.

Smerdyakov

Dreadful-sounding name, I know. I think it means 'stinking one'. (Alistair tells me that 'smert' is also Russian for 'death'.) This Smerdyakov is the illegitimate son of a poor deranged woman called Lisaveta, who used to hang round the town. No one knows who got her with child, but the unspeakable Karamazov senior is a prime candidate, which would make Smerdyakov the fourth Karamazov brother. (It's a bit like the Marx brothers: you think there are only three and suddenly a fourth one pops up, or even a fifth.)

Smerdyakov is more than a little sinister. He hints to Ivan that if Ivan were to go away, then Mitya might feel free to kill their father. What about Smerdyakov himself? He was the only other person around that night but he couldn't have done the deed because he was in *status epilepticus* at the time. Or was he just faking it? I shall say no more for fear of spoiling the suspense for you. I shall just note that Smerdyakov is highly intelligent and second only to Ivan in theological argument. His demolition of the case for admiring martyrdom (Book 3, Chapter 7) is masterly and extremely funny. Which reminds me, it's time we had a section on religion.

Religious controversies: does God exist?

In addition to some colourful characters and a thrilling crime story, Dostoyevsky also supplies a bonus in the form of a series of debates about religion. The existence or otherwise of a divine order is very important to the Karamazovs: they feel that if there is no God then 'anything is permitted' and it is quite OK to murder your old man if he is interfering with your plans. Dostoyevsky himself believed fervently in God and the Orthodox Church; but he obviously had painful doubts which he wrestled with, just like his fictional creations. And, very sportingly, he seems to have put the most eloquent arguments in the mouth of Ivan the unbeliever (although he too has tremendous spiritual struggles which, in the end, seem to drive him to madness).

In Book 5, Ivan and Alyosha meet in an inn and have a long conversation about God. As I have indicated, Ivan does most of the talking while Alyosha (and the rest of us) listen open-mouthed. Ivan starts by talking about all the suffering in God's world and in particular the suffering of children. He gives some heart-rending accounts of atrocities to children which he says have happened recently in Russia. The modern reader is only too painfully aware that similar things are still happening today, and not just in Russia. Finally, Ivan says that, even if God one day reveals his purpose and explains his reasons, it will still not be worth the price of one little child's suffering. He is willing to accept that God exists but, for Ivan, the price of belonging to God's world is too high: 'It's not that I don't accept God, Alyosha. I'm just, with the utmost respect, handing Him back my ticket'.

After returning his ticket, Ivan goes on to relate to his brother a story he has composed called 'The Legend of the Grand Inquisitor'. Yes, this is the one, perhaps the most famous episode in the whole novel and one of the most stunning chapters in World Literature. Briefly, what happens in Ivan's 'legend' is that Jesus comes back to earth in sixteenth-century Seville, at the height of the Spanish Inquisition when, nearly every day, heretics were being burned to death by the Church. The crowd recognise Him at once as He walks among them. He starts to bless them and some are healed by touching His garments. Then, the Grand Inquisitor appears in the Square. He is an old man of 90, 'tall and erect with a withered face and sunken eyes which, however, still glint with a fiery gleam'.

The confrontation between these two is really dramatic and the way Ivan tells it will have you transfixed with nervous anticipation and wonder. What does the Inquisitor do? He has Jesus arrested! In the evening he comes to Jesus's cell and tells Him 'you are not wanted here'. The gist of his argument is that Jesus had His chance 15 centuries earlier and He blew it. The standard

He set for humanity was just impossibly high. He should have listened to the devil and given people bread and miracles instead of burdening them with the unwanted gift of free will. Well, says the Inquisitor, we have taken over now. We feed them and promise them forgiveness and salvation in return for obedience. So get out of here and if you show your face again I'll have you burned as a heretic.

And what does Christ say? Not a word. He simply kisses the Grand Inquisitor on the lips and disappears into the back streets, never to be seen again. As for the Inquisitor: 'the kiss glows in his heart but the old man sticks to his idea'.

Whether all this high-intensity theology is good for you I am not certain. It will certainly make a powerful impression and you may have to lie down in a darkened room for a few hours afterwards. The last time you took part in this sort of debate was probably when you were a student: about the same age as the Karamazov boys. But now we must return to the story, because today is the opening of the Great Karamazov Murder Trial and the whole town is buzzing with excitement.

The courtroom drama

This is like a John Grisham novel only about a hundred times better-written. The trial is described by our faithful friend, the anonymous narrator, who knows all the personalities and can tell you all the gossip. He sets the scene brilliantly and, as you read, you feel as if you are sitting in the crowded courtroom, looking around at all the faces and listening eagerly as he points people out to you. Most of the men in the public gallery are hoping and expecting to see Mitya convicted. But the ladies (of whom there are a great many) are 'overwhelmingly on his side and hoping for an acquittal'. The case has attracted attention all over Russia and there are many eminent visitors. The local public prosecutor is hoping that a success in this case will revive his dwindling reputation. But he is up against the famous Fetyukovich, a distinguished lawyer from St Petersburg who has been sufficiently interested in the case to come down to town to defend Mitya.

I won't give you all the details of the trial, but I promise you that it is full of incidents and surprises. Mitya's two lady friends make passionate interventions, neither of which does him much good. The prosecutor displays the known facts with deadly precision. Mitya has been heard to shout that he will kill his father (it is perfectly true, we have heard him ourselves). There are also plenty of witnesses ready to testify that he was desperate to get his hands on some money on the day before the murder. And then he was seen, shortly afterwards, covered with blood and throwing around rainbow-coloured 100 rouble notes. Surely the case is open and shut. But then the famous counsel from Petersburg stands up and starts to discredit all the witnesses. And what about Smerdyakov, the number two suspect? He is said to have confessed to the murder, but we only have Ivan's word for it. Both counsels make persuasive use of psychology and imagination in their appeals to the jury.

Is Mitya guilty or not? And what are those solid fellow citizens on the jury thinking? Will he be convicted or acquitted? Well, obviously, I'm not going to spoil it by telling you. In any case, I am not sure I can remember: the writing is so fiendishly clever that a few days after I finish the book I find that I am no longer quite sure what happened in that courtroom and I have to read it again.

Alyosha and the schoolboys

The last part of the book, the epilogue, is largely devoted to Alyosha and some young schoolboys he has befriended. There are two earlier sections (Books 5 and 10) devoted to this little group and in particular to the rather pathetic family of one of them. This boy is called Ilyusha (which sounds a bit like Alyosha) and sadly he dies of some unnamed disease, probably tuberculosis. In the last chapter, Alyosha and the other boys attend Ilyusha's funeral and Alyosha urges them all to 'be first, and above all, kind and then honest and then – don't let us forget each other'. This is quite moving and Alyosha is such a decent fellow you have to like him. But I have to say that I think the sections of the book which deal with the schoolboys are the least successful. Dostoyevsky was very interested in the way children are brought up and these episodes were clearly of great importance to him. Perhaps they would have been properly developed if he had lived to write the definitive story of Alyosha in *Karamazov 2*. We shall never know.

I shall leave you with a final tip: on no account miss the chapter called 'Cana of Galilee' (Book 7, Chapter 4). Dostoyevsky declared that it was possibly the most important in the novel. It is about the way you feel when your heart has been full of pain and conflict and then, all at once, someone speaks to you as if in a dream and, suddenly, everything makes sense, you run outside and gaze rapturously at the star-studded heavens and fling yourself down to embrace and kiss the earth. It is really inspiring. And very Russian.

The text

The Brothers Karamazov by Fyodor Dostoyevsky was first published in 1880. It is available in paperback in a number of English translations. The translation by David Magarshack was first published in 1958 by Penguin Books Ltd, London. Extracts reproduced by permission of Penguin Books Ltd.

10

Tess of the d'Urbervilles

by Thomas Hardy

Today we are off to the West Country: to the chalk ridges and the gentle green valleys of Wessex. Our guide is Mr Thomas Hardy (1848–1928) and Wessex is his name for the area of Somerset, Hampshire and especially Dorset, in which he set his novels. Our heroine is called Tess Durbeyfield and just why she should be (ironically) called 'of the d'Urbervilles' we shall shortly discover. Tess is a lovely girl and you will feel for her as you would for your own daughter, as no doubt Hardy did when he created her. So it is a little difficult to understand why he gave her such a hard time and such a tragic, short life. Reading Tess can be a painful experience, although there are moments of happiness and long passages of great beauty as Hardy magically brings the landscape to life so you can hear the birds and bees, smell the flowers and feel the warm summer breeze on your cheek. But before I get carried away, let's open *Tess of the d'Urbervilles* at Chapter 1 and see how it begins.

The story opens with a description of a middle-aged man walking back to his village (in Wessex, of course) from a visit to the nearby town of Shaston. On the way he meets an elderly parson on horseback who surprises him by addressing him as 'Sir John'. In fact, he's not a knight, he's a poor 'haggler' (which means a kind of pedlar who trudges around selling produce) and he's our heroine's Dad (we'll meet her very soon). It turns out the old parson is a bit of an amateur genealogist and he's discovered that the Durbeyfields are descended from an aristocratic family called d'Urberville who came over with William the Conqueror. Of course, the family have long since lost all their money and prestige and so the connection doesn't mean very much in practical terms. But Jack Durbeyfield is a rather vain and self-deluding chap and he soon convinces himself (with the help of a few drinks) that a new life of money and leisure beckons him and his family.

Chapter 2 takes us to the village of Marlott in the Vale of Blackmoor, where the Durbeyfields live. Hardy gives us the first of many appealing descriptions of the countryside of his boyhood, which make you want to rush down there as soon as possible and enjoy it ('… for the most part untrodden as yet by tourist or landscape painter' he says – but that was in 1891). If you do wander down there you will certainly find the village of Marlott – but its real name is Marhull; Hardy changed all the names as if to distinguish real Wessex from the virtual Wessex of his imagination. Or possibly to make the places harder to find.

Anyway, when we arrive in Marlott, we find a May Day dance going on. All the young girls of the village are walking in procession, wearing white gowns and carrying a peeled willow wand and a bunch of white flowers. They are all pretty, but the one you really notice (with a nudge from Mr Hardy) is Tess Durbeyfield. She is the one with the large eyes, the deep red mouth and a pouting lower lip – and a red ribbon in her hair. How old is Tess? Probably barely 17; a young woman but in many ways still a child. 'For all her bouncing handsome womanliness, you could sometimes see her twelfth year in her cheeks or her ninth sparkling in her eyes; and even her fifth would flit over the curves of her mouth now and then.'

Someone else has noticed Tess as well. There are three young men 'of superior class', dressed for a walking tour, who stand surveying the scene. The girls start to dance with each other because their boyfriends haven't finished work yet. They invite the young men to dance with them and one of them agrees. His name is Angel Clare. He doesn't dance with Tess, but as he is leaving (called away by his more stand-offish brothers) their eyes meet, and they both seem to regret a lost opportunity. Well, readers, I have to tell you that this is one of the great lost opportunities of literature of which there are plenty in the works of our melancholy friend Mr Hardy. The thing is: if Tess and Angel had danced together that carefree day on Marlott village green their tragic story might have been a happy one. Mr Hardy knows that and he wants us to know it too. Life's a bitch and God is dead, he would say if he were with us today.

But don't let me start getting upset at this stage because I still have a long tale to unfold and it is time to meet the Durbeyfields at home and get to know our heroine a little better. Chapter 3 is a good place to draw a genogram of Tess's family. You will discover that she is the eldest of seven children (not counting the two who died in infancy). Dad, whom we've already met staggering home full of spurious family pride, is an amiable chap but not a very supportive father and a little too fond of the drink. Tess's mother, Joan, is also good-natured and takes care of the family as best she can. But Tess, at 17, is already having to take on a good deal of adult responsibility – watching out for her parents as well as the younger children. Our Tess is not just a simple country girl, she has reached the sixth standard in school, which must be around GCSE level, and she has been taught by a London-trained mistress. When I think of what she might have achieved with someone like you or me to guide her … but I mustn't go on like this. The younger children range from sister Lisa-Lu (12) through Abraham (9), the two younger girls (Hope and Modesty) to a boy of three and 'the baby'. Quite a responsibility for a teenager with two rather inadequate parents.

Now there is an interesting medical bit just here which I must tell you about because it has escaped the notice of all previous commentators. Mrs Durbeyfield tells Tess that father has been to see the doctor while he was in the town and there is 'fat round his heart'. She holds up her thumb and forefinger in the shape of a letter C and uses the other forefinger as a pointer; '"At the present moment," he says to your father, "your heart is enclosed all round there, and all round there: this space is still open, 'a says. As soon as it do meet, so" – Mrs Durbeyfield closed her fingers into a complete circle – "off you will go like a shadder Mr Durbeyfield, 'a says. You mid last ten years: you mid go off in ten months or ten days".'

Like me, you will instantly recognise this as an accurate description of the pathological anatomy and natural history of coronary artery disease! Mrs Durbeyfield thinks she is talking about fat round the heart but actually she is describing the gradual occlusion of a coronary artery by a C-shaped atherosclerotic plaque. We don't know if the doctor followed up his diagnosis with any healthy living advice – at any rate his patient didn't comply because he was off down the pub shortly after arriving home and giving the news to his wife. And who can blame him. I think we should follow him and as we stroll along I shall fill you in on what the local pubs are like, because you will need this information if we are going to spend some time in Marlott. Basically it is a long, straggling village with a pub at either end. There's the Pure Drop, which is more comfortable and fully licensed, but it's a long step from the Durbeyfield residence when you have a thirst on you. And besides, the beer is not as good as the brew at Rolliver's, which is conveniently located at our end of the village. The only problem about Rolliver's is that Mrs Rolliver doesn't actually have a licence to serve drink on the premises, so there's no lounge bar and customers have to sit in the upstairs bedroom on the bed, the chest of drawers or wherever they can find to squat. And if the authorities come round, Mrs R has to pretend she has just invited a few friends in for a private celebration. But no one thinks this is a problem. So it is to Rollivers' that Mr D has gone with his dodgy ticker and his newly acquired upper class lineage. Mrs D soon joins him and they talk to their friends about the d'Urberville connection. They learn that there is a lady called d'Urberville living not far away at Trantridge, who must be a rich relation, and the elder Durbeyfields hatch a plan to send Tess, their most presentable representative, to visit her ladyship and 'claim kinship'.

Tess isn't too keen on this plan but the events of the next 24 hours make her feel that she has to agree to it. Her father is due to convey a load of beehives to Casterbridge (Dorchester) in time for the market the following day. But he is not well enough for the trip and so Tess has to go in his place, taking her little brother,

Abraham, for company. The journey is such a long one that they have to start at 2 am. Both children are sleepy, having been roused after only a couple of hours in bed, but they set off on the rickety family cart drawn by Prince, the faithful old family horse. On the way, they have a rather poignant conversation. They look up at the stars, which Tess says are all worlds, a bit like the apples on their tree. Most are sound but a few are blighted, and they are unlucky enough to live on a blighted one (a very Hardyian view). Then they both fall asleep, the cart has a head-on collision with the morning mail cart and poor old Prince gets the shaft through his heart. With the death of the horse goes the family's means of support. Tess feels it was all her fault and that she had better make amends by agreeing to go off and introduce herself to the rich 'relatives'.

So off she goes, by foot and horse-drawn van across country to The Slopes, where Mrs d'Urberville has her seat. She is surprised to find that the buildings are all new and made of red brick. 'Everything looked like money.' We soon learn that the owners are not an old family at all: they are really called 'Stoke-d'Urberville', having added on the local d'Urberville name as a conceit when they moved into the region.

As Tess stands wondering what to do, a male voice says. 'Well, my beauty, what can I do for you?' The owner of the voice is a dark, handsome, moustachioed young man. Yes, this is Alec d'Urberville, the vile seducer and villain of the piece, introducing himself. Alec says his mother is an invalid and can't be seen at present. Soon he is laying on the charm and showing the bewildered Tess (who has no experience of this sort of offensive) around the gardens. In a memorable scene, he offers her a strawberry, making her take it directly into her mouth from his fingers (very erotic). Then he fills her basket with strawberries and stuffs her hat and her bosom full of roses before allowing her to go home. When her parents hear about this adventure they are thrilled – they can already see their daughter making a magnificent marriage into a wealthy family. Mr Durbeyfield is quite willing to overlook Alec's lack of genuine ancestry. He is even willing to sell his putative son-in-law the d'Urberville title.

And so, although she would much rather stay away from the obnoxious Alec, Tess finds herself persuaded to go back there and accept a job looking after old Mrs d'Urberville's poultry. It isn't long before the rascally Alec is up to his tricks again. He takes Tess for a downhill ride at breakneck speed (very symbolic) so that she will cling to him in fear for her life, and enforces a kiss on her burning cheek (which she instantly wipes clean). But there is no escape. On another ride with Tess, this time on a misty moonlit night, Alec pretends that they are lost in the woods. Tess falls asleep on the ground, while Alec searches for the road. Then he returns and, I'm sorry to say, has his dastardly way with her.

The next section or 'phase' is called 'Maiden no more'. When we meet her again, Tess has been with Alec for four months and is wrenching herself away to return to her family. Her mother is amazed to hear that she is not going to marry Alec. She certainly doesn't want to – although it's not clear that he has ever asked her. But she is pregnant. 'You ought to have been more careful ...' says her mother. And poor Tess replies: 'I was a child when I left this house four months ago. Why didn't you tell me there was danger in men-folk? Ladies know what to fend hands against, because they read novels that do tell them of these tricks; but I never had the chance of learning in that way, and you did not help me.'

The months pass and we find Tess working in the fields, breast-feeding her baby during the lunch break. Her fellow workers look at her with compassion and curiosity, remarking that it always happens to the pretty ones. The baby is a little boy, aptly named 'Sorrow' by his mother. And I'm sorry to have to tell you that he sickens and is clearly not long for this world. Heartbreaking little scenes follow in which the young mother, assisted by her awe-stricken brothers and sisters, baptises her baby just in time. The mean-spirited parson refuses him a Christian burial so Tess slips the sexton a shilling and buries her baby in a corner of the churchyard at night, with a bunch of flowers in a marmalade jar to mark his grave. Mr Hardy will move you to tears when you read this. He will also kindle your anger against injustice and inhumanity.

The next phase is more cheerful; so you can put down the Kleenex box – but make sure it stays within reach. A couple of years have passed and the 19-year-old Tess is off to seek her fortune in the Vale of the Great Dairies. This is a wondrous region of lush grassland, where, as the name suggests, the chief source of wealth is the milk of the cow. Tess becomes a milkmaid in the establishment of Dairyman Crick. She is welcomed by the other milkmaids, who are very friendly, although they can see that Tess is just a touch superior to them in background and education. She soon learns how to milk cows and we readers profit from her education as well. You see, each cow is different, some are easy, some are difficult, and you have to get to know them individually. There are similarities to general practice.

Now as luck would have it, there is also a young man working at the Crick dairy, a young gentleman who is intent on becoming a farmer. Yes, it is none other than Angel Clare, that same Angel who saw Tess with her friends on the village green and made the mistake of not asking her to dance. This time they do get acquainted and they start to fall in love. There are some wonderful descriptions of their early morning walks together through the misty fields before sunrise. The other milkmaids are in love with Angel too – he is something of a dreamboat. In one memorable scene, the girls are cut off by a flooded road and Angel undertakes to carry them through the water one by one. They are all fainting with love and desire as they wait their turn to be ferried across in his arms. But all are agreed that Tess (whose turn comes last) is the one he really wants to have his arms around. When this chapter was submitted for serialisation in the magazine *The Graphic*, the editor thought it was more than his readers could cope with. Hardy had to rewrite it and have Angel transport the girls in a wheelbarrow! Fortunately the original version was restored to us when the story was published in book form. Finally, Tess and Angel embrace in the milking parlour while Old Pretty, the cow, looks on disapprovingly and lifts her leg discontentedly.

As well she might, because there is a problem. Tess keeps telling Angel that, although she loves him, she can't marry him. But she can't bring herself to tell him about her unhappy experiences with Alec and about the baby. She feels sure that if she does so he won't want any more to do with her. From our perspective this seems a little strange. Surely a man like Angel won't be bothered that he's not the first? Especially as Tess was little more than a child when she was taken advantage of. It's true that Angel is the son of a clergyman of fairly rigid beliefs, but he has rejected all that and become a liberal intellectual. All the same, Tess is troubled and full of foreboding. She continues to hold back her acceptance until one day when they ride through the rain together, delivering milk to the station (this is the dawning of the modern age and the milk is bound for London). On that rainy ride (echoing the rides with Alec) Tess creeps close to Angel and soon they are kissing passionately. She decides she will marry him and writes to her mother, who replies, urging her not to breathe a word about her past. Sensible advice you might think, but Tess is so open and honest that she can't bear to deceive Angel. One day, she writes him a letter, telling him all about Alec and pushes it under his bedroom door. She waits, palpitating, for his response, but the next day he says nothing. It turns out that the letter was pushed under the carpet and he never saw it. After that terrible suspense and let-down she can't face another attempt: she agrees to his urgent requests to name the day and they get married. On the wedding evening they sit in front of the fire and agree to tell each other their past sins. Angel relates a few boyish adventures which Tess readily forgives. And then 'she entered on her story of her acquaintance with Alec d'Urberville and its results, murmuring the words without flinching, and with her eyelids drooping down'.

How does our young man take the news? Very, very badly, I'm afraid. For such a sensible, warm-hearted chap his reaction is quite unreasonable, especially to our present-day ears. Tess is no longer the same woman he thought he loved, he declares, but another woman in her shape. It is not a matter of forgiveness, he forgives all right, it wasn't her fault – but everything has changed. Something deep within him just can not bear the thought that another man has made love to her, has been intimately acquainted with her body. Yes, she is still his wife, but there's no question of their living together, they must part. Poor Tess, we grieve for her, she doesn't deserve this cruel and unreasonable treatment. Oh dear, and it was just what she feared. Why didn't she listen to her mother's advice? And then we, the modern readers, get quite upset and angry with young Angel. What the devil is the matter with the boy? Is this the result of his vicarage upbringing proving stronger than his more recent intellectual convictions? Is it some sort of snobbery which makes him feel that if a gent like him is going to marry a simple country girl she must be in absolutely mint condition? Are all men basically like this, full of irrational possessive jealousy? Or is it just Mr Hardy, gloomy old bugger, determined to show us how rotten life must be, even for his own beloved creation. Well, we can argue about this for ever (I nearly said until the cows come home). It is a great debate that will go on as long as people read and enjoy *Tess of the d'Urbervilles*.

But let us follow Tess, because we are naturally anxious to find out what will happen to her now, and very apprehensive. Angel gives Tess £50 and says he's off to Brazil to investigate the prospects for farming there. He says he may send for her but he makes no promises. On his way he encounters one of the other milkmaids, Tess's friend Izz. Impulsively he offers to take her to Brazil with him (the bad boy). He asks her if she loves him more than Tess does and she replies memorably: 'Nobody could love 'ee more than Tess did! She would have laid down her life for 'ee. I could do no more!' That brings him to his senses and he gallops off alone.

Now our heroine undergoes physical suffering to go with her spiritual agony. She needs to find work and there is no more milking. Instead she gets a job in a hard, stony part of Wessex called Flintcombe-Ash. The only work available is back-breaking toil grubbing up the roots of swedes with an instrument called a 'hacker'. After a few weeks of this, even her resilient spirit is near breaking. She decides to set off on another of her 15-mile cross-country walks to Angel's parents' vicarage to seek some news of him. When she arrives they are all at church. She feels too humiliated to return to the vicarage and tramps away, pausing at another village. She finds everyone gathered to listen to an open-air preacher who turns out to be Alec d'Urberville! How is this possible? Rather unconvincingly, Alec has undergone a dramatic religious conversion and is now an itinerant preacher or 'ranter'.

He recognises Tess and from this point on he follows her everywhere. She is still a good-looking girl and his old desire for her ignites strongly. Soon he has thrown off his recently acquired piety (it never really suited him) and is back in determined lecherous pursuit of our heroine. He even has the cheek to blame her for his 'backsliding'. Wherever Tess goes, in village, field or country lane, the demonic Alec seems to pop out from behind a tree and offer to solve all her problems. He is not a bit bothered to hear she is married and says she should leave her 'mule of a husband' and come to him. When he tries to put an arm round her waist, Tess smacks him across the mouth with the hard leather glove she wears for hacking swedes. Serves him right, the blackguard. But I'm afraid he is undeterred.

Months later, Angel finally returns, having had a pretty awful time in South America. He is thin and exhausted and has probably had malaria and various other tropical diseases. Serves him right too. Nevertheless, he has been thinking a good deal during his sufferings in exile and he has discovered that he really misses his Tess terribly. Those old panicky 'Oh my God, she's not really a virgin' feelings seem to have been burnt away by the equatorial sun.

But where has Tess gone? The trail leads to a seedy hotel in Sandbourne (alias Bournemouth, a modern upstart of a town which Hardy loathed and despised). There she is registered as Mrs d'Urberville, sharing a room with the repulsive Alec. When Angel finds her (dressed by Alec in fine clothes) he pleads for forgiveness and asks her to come away with him; but she cries: 'Too late, too late.' The words send a cold shiver down the reader's spine. It seems that Alec has told her that Angel will never come back and that she has agreed to be Alec's 'wife' instead. Angel staggers off aimlessly and Tess goes back in to Alec.

Now events move rapidly and remorselessly. The next chapter is like something out of Edgar Allen Poe. The landlady of the Herons Hotel (a nosy old person) overhears Tess's anguished cries as she tearfully upbraids Alec for deceiving her. There are some sharp words from him, followed by a rustle and a silence. Then the landlady sees a spot on the ceiling which grows and grows into a heart-shaped, red patch and then starts to drip. Blood. Tess has stabbed her tormentor with the carving knife and killed him.

She runs after Angel and, thank goodness, catches up with him. This is unbearably exciting. She tells him what has happened and they are reconciled. The lovers are united once more, although he is thin and gaunt and she is now a murderer on the run. They find refuge in a deserted mansion, where I'm glad to say they are allowed to have five days of happiness together. It was very decent of Mr Hardy to allow them five days, because knowing what he is like one would have been grateful for even 24 hours. Yes, they spend five days together and lie in each others' arms for five whole nights. Then their presence is discovered and they flee over the hills to Salisbury Plain, pausing for rest at Stonehenge. The exhausted Tess sleeps on one of the ancient stones, stretched out like a sacrificial victim while Angel stands guard. A black dot is seen approaching in the distance. Then another and another. As they get closer they are seen to be men. The cops have arrived to arrest Tess. Retribution has arrived and will not be denied.

Tess wakes and says: 'Have they come for me?', and she gives herself up without a struggle. In the final, short, desolate chapter we see Angel and Tess's sister Lisa-Lu watching as a black flag is raised outside Winchester Gaol. They have hanged our Tess. Does this have to happen? I can't help thinking that a good lawyer would have got her off and that a modern author would have devoted at least 100 pages to a dramatic account of the trial. Perhaps Angel himself would have conducted the defence after a quick cram course at law school. But no, we must remember that for Thomas Hardy there are no easy solutions to life's brutal realities. We are not allowed to give Tess a happy ending. But she lives on nevertheless in the minds of everyone who reads about her. I hope, if you haven't yet done so, that you too will meet Tess and spend some time with her and Angel amid the beauty and the harshness of Hardy's Wessex. Then the memory of Tess and her world will stay with you too.

About the author

Thomas Hardy was born in the village of Upper Bockhampton, near Dorchester, and spent most of his life in the county of Dorset. His father was a stonemason and Thomas was trained as an architect in London. During his student years he lost his religious faith. He returned to Dorset and began to write novels. His best-known books include *Far From the Madding Crowd, The Mayor of Casterbridge, Jude the Obscure* and, of course, *Tess*. He married Emma Gifford, with whom he endured a stressful marriage, but after her death he wrote some nice poems about her. When he was 74 he married his secretary, Florence Dugdale. He was greatly loved by his readers but attracted hostile review from the critics, who accused him of both pessimism and immorality. After *Jude* (which had a very rough reception) he gave up novel writing and concentrated on poetry. He ended up as a grand old man of English literature, loaded with honours. His heart was buried in the grave of his first wife (Emma) next to the tombs of his parents in Stinsford churchyard (Dorset). The rest of him is in Poets' Corner, Westminster Abbey.

The text

Tess of the d'Urbervilles by Thomas Hardy was first published in 1891. The Penguin Classics edition has notes by David Skelton and an introduction by A Alvarez.

11

The Life and Opinions of Tristram Shandy

by Laurence Sterne

For our next literary masterpiece we go back to the eighteenth century and a wonderful secret which I am eager to share with you. The secret is that, although *Tristram Shandy* was written a very long time ago and its style may seem a little archaic, once you begin reading it you will soon find that it is amazingly modern and accessible. It is also funny, entertaining, frequently indecent, heart-warming and thought provoking. It may also drive you crazy but that is a risk you are going to have to take. Where shall we start? I'll begin by telling you a little about the author.

About the author

Laurence Sterne was an obscure clergyman, born in Ireland in 1713, who acquired a country living in Coxwold in Yorkshire. He was very thin and suffered all his life from pulmonary tuberculosis, which eventually did for him. He was married, not very happily, and had a family. People who heard them said he preached good sermons. And that might have been all there was to say about Laurence, had he not started writing this extra-ordinary book in 1759, when he was 46. The first two volumes came out that year and he produced seven more in the next few years before the project finally ran out of steam. Later on he wrote a sort of travel book called *A Sentimental Journey* (also a great success), which was published a few months before his death in 1768.

If that was Laurence Sterne, who was Tristram Shandy? Tristram is Sterne's fictional alter ego and the book is a sort of spoof autobiography. But it is not like any other autobiography you have ever read, mainly because of the terrible struggles Tristram has in getting his story told. As he complains at one point, 'I have been at it these six weeks, making all the speed I possibly could – and am not yet born.' In fact, it is not until volume three (after a prolonged literary labour and a disastrous forceps delivery) that he finally emerges from the womb. The reason for this delay is that Tristram believes in beginning at the begin-ning and omitting none of the details. The details include every idea that occurs to him during the process of telling the story and all the associated ideas that these throw up. The author (whether he is Sterne or Tristram is not quite clear) also keeps stopping to engage the reader in conversation, which is one of the things which make you feel that, although the writer died over 200 years ago, he is alive and well, looking over your shoulder and reading your mind while you read his book. He keeps begging us to be patient with his all-inclusive style and to let him tell his story in his own way. (We family doctors have heard that before, somewhere.) And, like many of our patients, he goes in for lengthy digressions on all manner of subjects. Digressions are very important in this book and Sterne makes no apology for them. On the contrary, 'Digressions', he says 'incontestably are the sunshine, they are the life, the soul of reading; take them out of this book for instance and you may as well take the book along with them.'

I think that reading Tristram Shandy has changed my whole attitude to digressive patients. When somebody in the surgery starts off on a long and apparently irrelevant narration I remind myself that 'digressions are the sunshine' and I sit back and enjoy the story. It takes time but it may lead to the diagnosis. Just as often, it leads to a different kind of revelation about the patient or oneself or something or other. Whatever it is, I usually feel better for it. Isn't that strange? But I can see that I am in danger of losing the plot myself (the Shandy style is very infectious), so let's get back to the story.

Open the book

We shall open the book at Volume 1, page 1, and I am going to walk you gently through the first few chapters, because the style is a bit difficult to tune into at first and I don't want you to miss any of the hidden jokes. Once you have the hang of it (which you soon will, I promise) I shall merely point out a few signposts along the way, introduce you to the principal characters, say a few more words about the unique Shandeian style, and let you proceed at your own pace and in your own way. So let us begin, as Tristram does, at the moment of his own conception. What's this, you say: a sex scene in Chapter 1? I read it through just now and sex wasn't even mentioned! Let's read it over again:

> *I wish either my father or my mother, or indeed both of them, as they were in duty both equally bound to it, had minded what they were about when they begot me; had they duly considered how much depended upon what they were then doing: ... I am verily persuaded I should have made quite a different figure in the world.*

Tristram goes on to say that something he calls 'the animal spirits' are 'transfused from father to son' during the act of procreation. These animal spirits accompany the homunculus (he means the spermatozoon) and 'conduct him safe to the place designed for his reception'. Now it seems that if the couple are not concentrating fully on their pleasurable activity the animal spirits are dispersed, with disastrous consequences for the future welfare of the soul of the new person who is being created. This is only one of the strange biological notions held by Tristram (and his father). So what disturbed their concentration? Only this:

> 'Pray, my dear,' quoth my mother, 'have you not forgot to wind up the clock?' 'Good G**!' cried my father, taking care to moderate his voice at the same time, 'Did ever woman, since creation of the world, interrupt a man with such a silly question?' Pray what was your father saying? – Nothing.

And that is the end of Chapter 1. Tristram's father was 'saying' nothing because he was approaching his orgasm. Mrs Shandy, it seems, was not quite there with him.

We later learn (in Chapter 4) that Tristram's methodical father had adopted the habit of winding up the grandfather clock on the first Sunday night of every month: 'and had likewise gradually brought some other little family concernments to the same period, in order … to get them all out of the way at one time and be no more plagu'd and pestered with them the rest of the month'. One of the delights of Sterne's way of writing is that this sentence seems perfectly reasonable at first reading: and then you realise that making love to poor Mrs Shandy is one of the 'little family concernments' tidied away among all the rest. Fortunately she seems to have a very equable temperament.

In Chapter 5, Tristram records his birth and bemoans the misfortunes that have beset him ever since he was 'brought forth into this scurvy and disastrous world of ours'. (Most of these chapters are quite short: some are only half a page.) In Chapter 6, he cheers up a little and has a chat to the reader. You must have patience with me, he says, if you think I am proceeding slowly. I will tell you more about myself as we get to know each other better. We are still strangers to each other but I hope as we travel on we shall become friends, 'and as we jog on, either laugh with me, or at me, or in short do anything – only keep your temper'.

Midwives and hobby horses

Chapter 6 introduces the midwife who will play an important (although entirely unseen) role in Tristram's birth. We learn that she is established in practice as a result of the generosity of a local parson's wife. Somehow, this leads, via a longish digression about hobby horses (about which more later), to an account of the life of the local parson himself. He is called Yorick (like the late, lamented jester in *Hamlet*). Yorick makes an appearance in the plot later on and he is generally regarded as a portrait of Sterne himself. By this time Tristram has become so caught up in his digressions that he appears to have forgotten that he is supposed to be describing his own birth. Will he ever return to the main theme? There are further digressions which circle around it by way of the reasons why his mother was confined in the country and not in London, and whether babies may be baptised *in utero* if they are in imminent danger of death (it can be done with a syringe, but only if you are a Catholic). There is a detailed account of all this in French (not too difficult), which leads Mr Shandy (père) to the idea that it might save time and trouble to baptise all the homunculi (spermatozoa) in advance with *'une petite canulle'* inserted into … the appropriate place. Provided the father is not injured in the process, naturally.

That was Chapter 24. Suddenly in Chapter 25 we are back to the plot. We are in the parlour of Shandy Hall with Tristram's mother evidently in labour upstairs. 'I wonder what's all that noise and running backwards and forwards for, above stairs', says his father. He is talking to his brother, Tristram's Uncle Toby, whom I shall tell you more about in a minute. '"What can they be doing, brother?" – quoth my father, – "we can scarce hear ourselves talk". "I think", replied my Uncle Toby', but before he can voice his thoughts we are off on another philosophical digression. All this intellectual curiosity means that Mrs Shandy's labour is prolonged even further and the midwife is not sent for until well into Volume 2. I told you this would drive you crazy. However, Tristram is on hand in Chapter 21 to tell us that although he is frequently flying off on a digression he takes care that 'my main business does not stand still in my absence'. With that reassurance ringing in your ears you may now have a little rest while I tell you about some of the colourful characters in the Shandy family and household. And as they all play their part in the story it will give me a chance to fill you in on the story of Tristram's birth while he is preoccupied with his digressions.

Uncle Toby

Tristram's Uncle Toby is an old soldier, a veteran of Marlborough's campaigns against the French, which I remember vaguely from school history. He has had to retire from the army because, at the siege of Namur, he suffered a wound 'upon his groin' caused by the fall of a heavy stone from part of the town's defensive walls. As a result of this traumatic incident, Toby has become obsessed with sieges, projectiles and fortifications. He is abetted in this absorbing interest by his faithful retainer Corporal Trim, another retired soldier from his old regiment. At first Toby makes maps of all the sieges going on in the current wars (which he reads about in the papers). Then Corporal Trim hits on the idea of actually building scale models of each town that the British and their allies are besieging on the bowling green in Uncle Toby's back garden. The fortifications are copied exactly and then carefully breached and destroyed as reports reach England of another military triumph. This is Uncle Toby's famous 'hobby horse', about which his brother Walter (Tristram's father) can be very scathing. But Toby never takes offence. He is a wonderfully benign and gentle fellow who is easily moved to tears by the misfortunes of any fellow creature. In one celebrated passage, he even empathises with a fly that is buzzing round his nose at dinner time. Instead of swatting the fly, he carefully catches it and lets it out of the window. '"I'll not hurt thee", says my Uncle Toby, rising from his chair, and going across the room, with the fly in his hand – "I'll not hurt a hair of thy head: go," says he, lifting up the sash and opening his hand as he spoke, to let it escape, "go, poor devil, get thee gone, why should I hurt thee? This world surely is wide enough to hold both thee and me."' And if, as sometimes happens, Uncle Toby feels a little slighted or out of countenance (as may happen if his hobby horse is treated with disrespect), he restores himself to equanimity by simply whistling a few bars of 'Lillabulero'. It is not possible for me to represent this well-known tune in musical notation but it will be familiar to listeners to the BBC World Service as their much loved (and recently discarded) signature tune.

Returning to the parlour at Shandy Hall, where time remains suspended at the moment we left it, what *did* Uncle Toby think about all the noise and running about up stairs? '"I think," replied my Uncle Toby, taking ... his pipe from his mouth and striking the ashes out of it as he began his sentence, "I think," replied he, "it would not be amiss, brother, if we rung the bell."'

The bell is answered by Obadaiah, the Shandys' principal manservant. He informs them that the Mistress 'is taken very badly' and Mrs Shandy's maid (Susannah) has run off to fetch the midwife. This news annoys Tristram's father because he would much rather have his wife attended by the 'man-midwife', the eminent Dr Slop (whom I shall introduce shortly). Mr Shandy has great faith in Dr Slop's obstetric skills (he is the owner of a very up-to-date set of forceps); but Mrs Shandy unaccountably prefers the female practitioner.

Uncle Toby, in his innocence, is inclined to think this due to her modesty: '"My sister, I dare say," added he, "does not care to let a man come so near her ****."'

This statement astonishes Tristram's father. How can Toby know so little about women? 'Methinks ... you might at least know so much as the right end of a woman from the wrong.'

'Right end of a woman?' mutters poor Uncle Toby, 'I know no more which it is, than the man in the moon'. So his brother embarks on an explanation, making use of the science of analogy: '"Everything in this world," continued my father (filling a fresh pipe), "everything in this earthly world, my dear brother Toby, has two handles." "Not always," quoth my uncle Toby ...'. Alas, this fascinating discussion is never completed because there is a 'devil of a rap at the door', and the plot must, for once, continue.

Enter Dr Slop

Who is at the door? None other than Dr Slop, himself. And our medical man is in considerable disarray. It appears that Obadaiah, riding at a gallop at his master's bidding to summon Dr Slop to the case, has collided with the poor doctor (who was already on his way) and knocked him off his pony into the mud. 'Imagine yourself a little, squat, uncourtly figure of a Doctor Slop, of about four feet and a half perpendicular height, with a breadth of back, and a sesquipedality of belly, which might have done honour to a serjeant in the horse-guards.' Not only is Dr Slop an unprepossessing figure, he has come to the confinement unequipped. In his haste, he has left his new-invented forceps and all his other instruments hanging up 'in a green bays bag' between his two pistols at the head of his bed. Obadaiah will have to be sent to fetch them. But no matter. The two brothers and the doctor are very happy to settle down to some enjoyable philosophical discussions while they wait for the equipment to arrive. This occupies quite a lot of pages, and causes some concern for those of us who are worrying about how Tristram's mother is progressing in her so far unattended labour. For there is clearly no question of Tristram's father being at the bedside to hold her hand while there are pipes to be smoked and discussions to be had downstairs in the parlour.

The next person to arrive is Corporal Trim, Uncle Toby's comrade and batman. The corporal shares Uncle Toby's empathetic disposition and is also easily moved to tears. He gets particularly sad when he is reminded of his brother Tom who was arrested by the Spanish Inquisition and all because he married a Jew's widow who kept a sausage shop (could this be another digression waiting in store for us? You surmise correctly). I have already mentioned the corporal's devotion to Uncle Toby and his skill in recreating besieged cities in miniature on the bowling green. He also plays a crucial role in Uncle Toby's affair of the heart with Widow Wadman. Have I not mentioned her yet? I have so much to tell you about this book I am in danger of running into several volumes myself.

Uncle Toby and Widow Wadman

The story of Uncle Toby's *amours* is told in the last two volumes (8 and 9), although, chronologically, it precedes Tristram's birth. Mrs Wadman is a neighbour who is much taken with Uncle Toby's soldierly good looks and amiable disposition. She is eager to mount her campaign by laying siege to his heart (a method which this student of sieges will understand only too well). But, she is rather worried by the reports she has heard about 'the wound upon his groin'. What sort of a wound is it, she wonders. And what exactly is meant by his 'groin'. In what precise way does the wound impair his capacities? 'Was he able to mount a horse? Was motion bad for it?' Widow Wadman is desperate to find out before committing herself fully to her campaign.

Imagine her excitement, then, when Uncle Toby offers to show her exactly where he received the wound. She debates with herself whether it would be right for her to look at it and decides that she will. '"You shall lay your finger upon the place," said my uncle Toby. "I will not touch it," however, quoth Mrs Wadman to herself.' But before my readers get too excited about this scene and start thumbing through the book in premature search for it, I should prepare them for a deflation – and would remind them that Uncle Toby is a man who has not yet learned to tell the right from the wrong end of a woman.

A forceps delivery

Now that I have introduced you to Widow Wadman I think we should return to the parlour at Shandy Hall and catch up with what is going on. We shall find that delightful conversations about philosophy, religion and human nature are in full swing. Corporal Trim reads a long and interesting sermon (very relevant in times like ours), which has unaccountably dropped out of a book on engineering which was urgently needed for reference on another subject. There are also important discussions on obstetrics, because Mrs Shandy's travails upstairs (thank God the midwife has now arrived) are never entirely forgotten by the considerate gentlemen in the parlour. Dr Slop is eager to talk about recent advances in obstetric technique, although Uncle Toby cunningly manages to turn the subject to the war in Flanders and the science of fortification whenever possible. The 'green bays bag', containing Dr Slop's instruments eventually arrives, knotted tightly with strings to prevent them from jingling. But unfortunately the knots are so tight they are impossible to untie. The doctor has to cut them with a knife and manages to cut his own thumb at the same time. This makes him feel like cursing, and happily an excellent written curse (text by a bishop, no less) is promptly provided by Tristram's father. I need hardly tell you it is in Latin and runs to a dozen pages. But there is an English translation and whether it is a cut finger or something less serious you will never again feel at a loss for a curse of sufficient power and devastation.

After delivering his curse and binding up his thumb, Dr Slop is soon ready for more digressions. And, eventually, to mount the stairs and apply the forceps. After that, all is quiet for a while until, suddenly, the company are disturbed by someone making a noise in the kitchen. Who can it be? It is Dr Slop, who, Obadaiah reports, is engaged on making a bridge. Uncle Toby immediately assumes that Dr Slop is thoughtfully helping to replace a damaged model bridge on the bowling green. However, it turns out that he is trying to make a bridge for baby Tristram's nose out of 'a piece of cotton and a thin piece of whale bone out of Susannah's stays'. Yes, Tristram has at last entered the world; but his poor little nose has been crushed as flat as a pancake by Dr Slop's clumsy application of the forceps. On receiving this dismal news Mr Shandy retires to his room and collapses on his bed in dismay. For him, this is only the latest in a series of calamities.

The naming of Tristram

You will remember the episode of the clock-winding reminder which disrupted the flow of animal spirits during Tristram's conception? That was the first. Mr Shandy has other deeply held beliefs about prenatal influences on the intellectual and spiritual development of the infant. In his view, the baby should be born breech first (to prevent harmful compression of the cerebellum) and should have a long nose (for reasons which I can't possibly go into now but you will find them fully set out in the latter part of Volume 3). So things look bad for Tristram's future development on all these counts. Only a good christening can mitigate these disasters; for Mr Shandy believes that the right choice of name is another vital factor determining an individual's success or failure in life.

'Trismegistus' is an excellent name it seems, full of promise. Whereas 'Tristram' is among the worst that a child could possibly have to bear the burden of. I think you might be able to guess the sort of thing that might go wrong here, but I will leave you to find and relish the details for yourselves.

We have now reached Volume 4 and young Tristram, although christened, is still incapable of speech. We have heard quite a lot of his opinions, but how much more of his life story is going to be revealed to us? One or two more rites of passage will be described (including his accidental circumcision) and we eavesdrop on a bedtime marital conversation in which the Shandy parents discuss their son's future. But the rest of his life, between acquiring his first pair of breeches and beginning to write his book, remains hidden. So, just what kind of autobiography do we have here?

More about the way the book is written

Reading this book is more than just listening to a story – it is a conversational journey in the company of a witty and brilliant man who died 232 years ago but is still very much alive. The story of Tristram's birth and the adventures of his Uncle Toby might have been told in a straightforward, linear manner and they would still have been very entertaining. I have no doubt that some of my readers who are uncomfortable with 'modernist' practices would have preferred it that way. But that is not what Sterne is about. He has lots of speculative and philosophical notions that he wants to explore (and send up) and he sees no reason why they shouldn't be part of the book as well. He is such a good talker that, if you are sitting comfortably in the parlour with him, it doesn't really matter how many times he interrupts his story to whisk you off on a digression. It seems that everything he says reminds him of something else which he absolutely has to tell you about, and he does it with such charm that you can't resist. I think we all have friends (and patients) who are a bit like that and sometimes they irritate the hell out of you. But in the end you forgive them and you let them continue as, irrepressibly, they must.

Another of Sterne's tricks is frequently to buttonhole the reader and engage him in conversation about how the book is progressing. He apologises for the slow pace of the story and the frequency of the digressions. He craves our sympathy for the enormous hardship he is undergoing in writing a life story in which events (or at any rate thoughts) are proceeding faster than he can get them down. He is concerned about our welfare too. At the end of Volume 4: 'The thing I have to ask is, how you feel your heads? My own akes dismally.'

For those who appreciate chapters and can't be doing with a long, unbroken narrative, Sterne provides much to enjoy. He is a real virtuoso of the art of chaptering. Some chapters are of normal length, but many are less than a page and some only a couple of lines. Two chapters are represented by blank pages (to be filled in later on when you had forgotten all about them). He also tries to cope with the constant flow of his own ideas by promising to deal with certain topics later on in specially designated chapters (rather like making 'Things to do' lists). So, for instance, we are promised chapters on chambermaids, knots, buttonholes, whiskers, *things* and long noses. There is even to be a chapter on chapters when he has time and space to fit it in. Some of these promises are fulfilled, while others languish. Then there are the strange pages and eccentric drawings. One page is black (in mourning for the death of Parson Yorick) and another is elegantly marbled (I don't know why, but someone will tell me). On one page there is a graphic representation of the progress of the story in each volume with the digressions shown as so many loops and wiggles. Indiscreet, whispered phrases are rendered in asterisks for the reader to fill in. I do hope you like this sort of nonsense.

How to read Tristram Shandy

Begin at the beginning. Read a little at a time. If you don't understand something, read it again. If you still don't understand it, move on and come back to it another time. Enjoy the conversations with your new friend Mr Sterne. Delight in the obstetric details attending Tristram's birth. Smoke (or smoak) a pipe with genial Uncle Toby. Let him tell you all about the prodigious armies they had in Flanders and show you the fortifications on the bowling green. Hold your breath as the Widow Wadman stalks him to within his very sentry box. On your first reading, you may skip some of the more abstruse digressions (but you must read every word of the Curse of Ernulphus, or *my* curse will be upon you). Otherwise, just read it gently at your own pace and in your own way. Keep reading it. Keep it by your bedside. Let the sunshine of digressions warm you into a good humour whenever you pick it up. 'True Shandeism, think what you will against it, opens the heart and lungs, and like all those affections which partake of its nature, it forces the blood and other vital fluids of the body to run freely through its channels, and makes the wheel of life run long and cheerfully round.'

The text

The Life and Opinions of Tristram Shandy, Gentleman by Laurence Sterne, was first published in 1759–67. Available in Penguin (edited and provided with especially useful notes by Graham Petrie) or Oxford University Press paperbacks.

Postscript: 'Seventh Heaven' by Alistair Stead

It might be thought apt that my supplement to John's introductory comments on *Tristram Shandy* should pivot principally on a gap, since Sterne repeatedly draws playful, often indecent, attention to various holes and crevices in his story and, according to taste, entertains or infuriates the reader with his virtuoso display of discontinuities, interruptions and breakings-off. So, where is comment on Volume 7? In what sense is this part of the book a gap itself, through which we can see – more clearly than usual – what, as they say, is up?

Now the Marquis de Sade once claimed that knowledge for writing fiction could be got 'only through misfortune and travel'. So it was for Sterne. John does credit to the muse of misfortune in pointing out the fun to be had from contemplation of Tristram as mangled child and bungling author, but the parts of the book on which he concentrates are, broadly speaking, domestic scenes where travel is represented by modest or trivial excursions. It is more important to notice that Tristram asks us to see life as a journey, and both writing and reading as voyages out. For the incurably digressive Sterne (or Tristram?), however, getting on with life or story tends to involve lots of regression or wandering from the straight and narrow. In this book, a major destination for the storyteller as traveller is to get to a promised recounting of the amours of Uncle Toby. Now, up to a point, this promise is kept (it depends on how you define 'amours' and whether you think the book is really finished off) and this account, given in the last two volumes (8 and 9), represents a kind of climax to Tristram's oddball autobiography and a proper tribute to the most humane influence on the narrator's disappointing life. To build to this anti-climactic climax (for just as Uncle Toby doesn't yield his virginity to Widow Wadman, Tristram doesn't appear to complete his life story or to gratify his sexual appetite), the narrator holds back from the finale, delaying it mightily by introducing a volume-long digression. He even draws attention to this in his epigraph to Volume 7. Translated from Pliny's Latin, it says: 'For this is no digression from it, but the thing itself.' Some critics see this as typical irony, but to me it is, in a sense, the truth. I wouldn't go so far as to say, like one critic (Douglas Brooks), that the seventh volume is therefore 'the real core of the book', for in an eccentric design there can be no core (centre) and reality is as kaleidoscopic as this book itself. But, if we look for some substantial reflection in *Tristram Shandy* of the generative impulse of travel, we shall find it in this seventh volume, where the digression is composed of a breathless travelogue, with Tristram's excursion to France mirroring closely what Sterne had just undertaken after he had seen the publication of the first six volumes. What is curious about this is that in the tale so far Tristram has largely been represented as either non-existent (he has not been born when Toby, in the climax, is assailed by the randy Widow) or a mere child (clumsily delivered, ineptly christened and accidentally circumcised). Only by implication (as the intrusive writer) or in fleeting revelations (as the wistful lover) are we conscious of the hero as an adult. Yet here, at last, we encounter the full-grown, almost full-frontal man, bent on travel and drawn to amorous adventure, and, like Sterne himself, seeking to escape from the fatal pulmonary tuberculosis which dogs him into new scenes and fresh company. As Sterne's dedication to Mr Pitt, which he added to the second edition of the first two volumes, declared: 'I live in a constant endeavour to fence against the infirmities of ill-health, and other evils of life, by mirth.' In this volume, it is easiest to recognise the human impulse behind the writing of this crazy masterpiece: the need to keep 'the spleen' at bay, the early-diagnosed consumptive's desperate defiance of his imminent death, through humour – and a kind of perpetual motion. The hectic pace of the prose, the excited rhythms, embody this escapism, although the melancholy source of it never impedes the flow, too, of whimsicality and bawdy. Thus this volume gives us our best glimpse of his 'seventh heaven' in a potentially therapeutic pastoral climax, where Tristram exchanges his dance of death for participation in a rustic round dance and for an ardent response to the singing by an amiable country girl of 'Viva la Joia! Fidon la Tristessa!' ('Long live Joy! Fie on Sadness').

This point can be reinforced if you like by following Douglas Brooks's lead[1] and entertaining the idea that Sterne was familiar with and prepared to exploit, however ambivalently, the ancient system of numerological symbolism (among other strange lore with which he toyed). Tristram in Volume 7, then, is attempting to fly from Saturn, the planet whose number is 7. It is the planet, associated with melancholy and mortality, which (mis)ruled over his birth. Tristram has been bound to this lord of sadness (*tristitia*) ever since his mismanaged christening, to the chagrin of a father who sees names as fatally significant. Seventh heaven, therefore, may be remission, temporary reprieve or safe haven from the inevitable, from this other, malign seven. You will see that it is evoked in Sterne's sporadically rhapsodic mode, yielding a moving impression of a precious transient joyfulness which elsewhere in the novel comes across in the more celebrated hilarious forms of farce, caricature, wordplay and parody.

Reference

1   Brooks D (1973) *Number and Pattern in the Eighteenth-Century Novel.*

12

The sonnets of William Shakespeare and John Donne

Oliver Samuel

Shakespeare

My discovery of Shakespeare may not surprise you, but at the time, it amazed me. I knew about and enjoyed the plays, but one day, when I was a student looking for an excuse not to go back to the dissecting room, I found a copy of his sonnets on a bookstall down on the quays in Dublin. This was a time when I was developing a burgeoning interest in poetry. My family had often played doggerel games during rainy days on holiday. We used to compete at writing verse in some of the more impossibly rigid court conventions – you should just read my triolets – so I knew about the technical structure of a sonnet. But suddenly there were these wonderful poems that carried the contents along in a way that prose could never reach. The technical structure was all there, but you hardly noticed, for the language and the passion swept everything else aside.

It was here that I began to feel the potency of real poetry for the first time; the way it can convey such emotional power within such a short span and release the imagination beyond the simple limits of the printed page. Curiously too, the rigid way a sonnet is constructed has a kind of liberation for the reader. Just as music is in rhythm and key, a sonnet carries its structure as a reassuring certainty, focusing attention all the more sharply on the contents. Just to remind you about the rules, a sonnet is a poem of 14 lines, each of which has ten syllables. The last six lines show a change of mood or reflect in a different way on the content of the first eight lines. In the Shakespearean form, the last two lines (which rhyme together) present yet another theme, or at least the summing up of what the poem is all about.

Of course, at the time the sonnets arrived, I was a spotty adolescent full of churned up emotions anyway, so that discovering passion and distress could be expressed with such ineffable skill was doubly amazing. 'Shall I compare thee to a summer's day' for me still conjures up the sunshine of June in College Park – the girls in light summer dresses and entwined couples under the trees. I only found out years later that this particular poem is actually addressed to a very pretty young man. What really struck me then and still does now is the range and variety of passionate ideas that Will managed to fit within the constraints of formal poesy. His sonnets read not so much constrained as enhanced by the totally predictable shape, rhyming scheme and rhythm, in which new ideas are created and blossom.

Now you do need to know that they were probably produced initially to please his sponsor, who was almost certainly gay. The first 126 sonnets are all addressed to a beautiful youth. The first ones all inveigh against him continuing to be unmarried. There is more than a hint of passion about them. Then in the last section the poems are written to an anonymous dark lady. There has been speculation about who the people were, but that all seems secondary to the quality – and quantity – of the verse. I wonder if Shakespeare wrote a sonnet every morning in the same way that some people tackle a crossword.

Originally I used to read the poems singly, just happening on one wherever the book opened. But now I prefer to read them in sequence, for they are thematic, with one sonnet leading to ideas in the next. This allows themes to develop and for some of the slightly less obvious ones to find their place in the ongoing courtly wooing of a wealthy and obviously pretty unpredictable sponsor. The later sonnets are wondrously romantic, but by no means sloppy. They voice plenty of criticism and resentment and every other emotion you can imagine.

For the most part I read poetry in bed, but I have had to ration myself, for I get caught up and have to keep on reading. I hope you find them as entrancing. Incidentally, I am currently using the Penguin edition, which has the text transliterated into modern spelling and provides an excellent introduction and running notes on each poem, just in case you are not quite up to scratch with Shakespearean naughty words. (Surely you know what 'will' means – yes over the years it has grown into 'willy'!)

My sense is that Shakespeare's sonnets are so tightly written that not even a comma can be changed without puncturing the magic and collapsing everything. What skill and what a joy that we still have these wondrous poems to savour. Have a look at one now and try to see if you can alter a single word and still keep the elegant consistency of the composition.

> When in disgrace with fortune and men's eyes,
> I all alone beweep my outcast state,
> And trouble deaf heaven with my bootless cries,
> And look upon myself and curse my fate,
> Wishing me like to one more rich in hope,
> Featured like him, like him with friends possessed,
> Desiring this man's art, and that man's scope,
> With what I most enjoy contented least;
> Yet in these thoughts almost myself despising,
> Haply I think on thee, – and then my state,
> Like to the lark at break of day arising
> From sullen earth, sing hymns at heaven's gate;
> For thy sweet love remembered such wealth brings
> That then I scorn to change my state with kings.

What is so extraordinary about the sonnets is their creativity: the range of ideas and situations that are conjured up. It is true that love is a recurring theme – thank God for that – but they scale from birth to death and there is never a hint of repetition. Such is their creative power that had Shakespeare never touched a play, then these alone would surely have ensured his literate im-mortality. Here are two more, that pun outrageously on the poet's name, just to set you wondering about their range.

Whoever hath her wish, thou hast the Will,
And Will to boot and Will in overplus;
More than enough am I that vex thee still,
To thy sweet will making additions thus.
Wilt thou, whose will is large and spacious,
Not once vouchsafe to hide my will in thine?
Shall will in others seem right gracious,
And in my will no fair acceptance shine?
The sea, all water, yet receives rain still
And in abundance addeth to its store;
As thou being rich in Will add to thy Will
One will of mine, to make thy large Will more.
Let 'no' unkind no fair beseachers kill;
Let all but one, and me in that one Will.

Or perhaps the next one did the job rather better.

If thy soul check thee that I come so near,
Swear to thy blind soul that I was thy will,
And will, thy soul knows, is admitted there;
Thus far for love my love-suit, sweet, fulfil.
Will will fulfill the treasure of thy love,
Ay, fill it full with wills, and my will one.
In things of great receipt with ease we prove
Among a number one is reckoned none.
Then in the number let me pass untold,
Though in thy store's account I one must be;
For nothing hold me, so it please thee hold
That nothing me, a something, sweet, to thee.
Make but my name thy love, and love that still,
And then thou lov'st me for my name is Will.

And to think that he just churned these poems out week after week, probably during a time that the theatres in London were closed during an outbreak of the plague. Wow.

John Donne

Well if I have managed to stir your interest in reading such marvellous stuff, let me acknowledge that, despite his reputation, I only really came to read my next poet very recently. I found the Penguin edition of *The Complete Poems of John Donne* by chance and thought that, although I had met Donne in short quotations, I had never had a real go at reading him properly. So a modest investment led to a slow and charming journey with this extraordinary man. Let me tell you a little about him.

About the author

John Donne was born in 1572, the third of six children. His father, a merchant, died when he was four. His mother was a staunch Roman Catholic – one of her brothers was exiled for being a Jesuit. She remarried Dr John Syminge, who later became President of the Royal College of Physicians and probably practised at Barts. When John Donne was 20 he was admitted to Lincoln's Inn and four years later he sailed from Plymouth as a gentleman adventurer under Walter Raleigh, to capture and loot Cadiz. Four years later he entered the service of Sir Thomas Egerton, Lord Keeper of England. In 1601, he entered Parliament as MP for Brackley and next year secretly married Sir Thomas's niece. When this was discovered he was sacked from his position and put (briefly) in the Fleet prison by his outraged father-in-law. I wonder if his proposal of marriage succeeded against obvious parental disapproval because of the amusing subtlety of his poetry. Do you think wooing with something like this might have helped?

> When I am dead, and doctors know not why,
> And my friends' curiosity
> Will have me cut up to survey each part,
> When they shall find your picture in my heart,
> You think a sudden damp of love
> Will through all the senses move,
> And work on them as me, and so prefer
> Your murder, to the name of massacre.

After some travelling and the birth of three children, he failed to get a job at Court, but he had made some important friends. The Countess of Bedford became godmother to his latest daughter and to her he wrote many elegant elegies. From 1607 onwards he tried unsuccessfully to find employment. In 1611, his sixth child was born and he joined Sir Robert Drury, travelling on the continent while his wife stayed with family on the Isle of Wight. By 1614 he was MP for Taunton, his elder daughter died and he continued to apply unsuccessfully for work. So in 1615, apparently for want of a better job, he was ordained as priest and was appointed deacon at St Paul's and made royal chaplain and (by royal command) received an honorary DD from Cambridge! Two years later his wife died. In the following years he was preaching all over Europe, often to royalty. In 1621, he was elected Dean of St Paul's, then was appointed judge in the Court of Delegates and spent the following years preaching and hearing cases in the ecclesiastical courts. He was preacher at King James' lying in state and to Charles I. In 1631, his mother died aged 83 and he died later the same year.

He published many sermons, some prose and a flood of poetry. Much of this was designed to butter up prospective employers or to heap praise on one of his sponsors, but that was far from all. He wrote witty, wicked, religious and profane verse with a marvellous range of styles. Often he produced new rhythms, internal rhymes and often too, he stayed conventional. He was just creative. How about this:

The Computation
For the first twenty years, since yesterday,
I scarce believed, thou couldst be gone away,
For forty more, I fed on favours past,
And forty on hopes, that thou wouldst, they might last.
Tears drowned one hundred, and sighs blew out two,
A thousand, I did neither think, nor do,
Or not divide, all being one thought of you;
Or in a thousand more, forgot that too.
Yet call not this long life; but think I
Am, by being dead, immortal can ghosts die?

Or try this one:

> Mark but this flea, and mark in this,
> How little that which thou deny'st me is;
> Me it sucked first, and sucks thee,
> And in this flea, our two bloods mingled be;
> Confess it, this cannot be said
> A sin, or shame, or loss of maidenhead.
> Yet this enjoys before it woo,
> And pampered swells with one blood made of two,
> And this alas, is more than we would do.

That is just the first verse, and he keeps up originality and persistence to the end of the poem. You really have to read it right through to get the gist of every twist and turn.

John Donne had a view of doctors that sounds embarrassingly similar to that of a Secretary of State for Health, although he expressed himself with rather greater elegance.

> The Doctors
> The sacred academe above
> Of Doctors, whose pains have unclasped, and taught
> Both books of life to us (for love
> To know thy Scriptures tells us, we are wrought
> In thy other book) pray for us there
> That what they have misdone
> Or mis-said, we to that may not adhere;
> Their zeal may be our sin. Lord let us run
> Mean ways, and call them stars, but not the sun.

What would you do if you received the following note of complaint that you hadn't written recently? The record does not show if there was a response, but I am sure it would be hard to stay in the same class.

> To Mr. R. W.
> Zealously my Muse doth salute all thee
> Inquiring of that mystic trinity
> Whereof thou and all to whom heavens do infuse
> Like fire, are made; thy body, mind and Muse.
> Doth thou recover sickness, or prevent?

Or is thy mind travailed with discontent?
Or art thou parted from the world and me,
In a good scorn of the world's vanity?
Or is thy devout Muse retired to sing
Upon her tender elegiac string?
Our minds part not, join then thy Muse with mine
For mine is barren thus divorced from thine.

Donne is probably best know for his religious poetry – the Holy Sonnets – but the elegies written to important people and the memorial poetry are all brilliant. Many of these works are quite long and you have to read them to appreciate the power of his imagination and the complete control with which he used the written word. But I cannot really illustrate that here. You need the full text. So, as I started with Shakespeare's sonnets, here to finish is a sonnet written by Donne to another friend, Mr T. W. about the inadequacy of his words.

Haste thee harsh verse as thy lame measure
Will give thee leave, to him, my pain and pleasure.
I have given thee, and yet thou art too weak,
Feet, and a reasoning soul and tongue to speak.
Plead for me, and so by thine and my labour,
I am thy Creator, thou my Saviour.
Tell him, all questions, which men have defended
Both of the place and pains of hell, are ended;
And 'tis decreed our hell is but privation
Of him, at least in this earth's habitation:
And 'tis where I am, where in every street
Infections follow, overtake, and meet:
Live I or die, by you my love is sent,
And you're my pawns, or else my testament.

The texts

William Shakespeare: The Sonnets and A Lover's Complaint (1986) John Kerrigan (ed). Penguin Books, Harmondsworth.

John Donne: The Complete English Poems (1971) AJ Smith (ed). Penguin Books, Harmondsworth.

13

A Country Doctor's Notebook and *The Master and Margarita*

by Mikhail Bulgakov

Tim Swanwick

Mikhail Bulgakov was born in Kiev in 1891. Although a doctor by training, he found his true vocation as a playwright and novelist. For the best part of his life, however, the writer was to be denied a voice. Bulgakov's plays failed to open and his novels, for the most part, remained unpublished. Indeed, his prose masterpiece *The Master and Margarita* did not appear in book form until 1973, more than 20 years after his death.

Like many leading Soviet artists of his day, Bulgakov had an intense and personal relationship with Josef Stalin. Many notable authors have explored the dictator's unhealthy preoccupation with the most creative of his Soviet citizens, most frequently in connection with the composer Dimitri Shostakovitch. The fact that the argument continues to rage over whether Shostakovitch was a subversive intellectual or a committed party member is testament to the uncertainty of those times, and indeed, the protective power of artistic ambiguity, perhaps something that music can provide in contrast to the bald directness of the written word.

In their dealings with Stalin, Shostakovitch and his fellow composer Sergei Prokofiev were lucky, or clever, or both. Both composers' works were frequently performed in their homeland during that time, if only once. But, for Bulgakov, things did not work out so well. Despite the relatively recent recognition that places him firmly in the pantheon of great Russian writers, only a tiny fraction of Bulgakov's output made it past the censors. For whatever reason, the writer was paralysed by Stalin, denied not only the opportunity to express himself, but also prevented from leaving the Soviet Union, despite requests made repeatedly to the Central Committee.

Bulgakov then, was a doctor – at least in the early days. It is perhaps not surprising that he chose medicine as a career; his stepfather and two of his uncles were doctors and although his main passion was for literature and the theatre, there were precedents in Chekhov and Veresayev. Chekhov in this typically candid quotation shows himself to be an early advocate of the portfolio career.

I feel more contented when I realise I have two professions not one. Medicine is my lawful wife and literature my mistress. When I grow weary of one, I pass the night with the other. Neither suffers from my infidelity.

In 1909, Bulgakov entered the University of Kiev to study medicine. By 1912, in a familiar storyline, he had failed his second year examinations. This was largely due to the disproportionate amount of time the young student had been spending with his girlfriend, Tatyana Nikolayevna Lappa. Despite family mis-givings, Bulgakov married Tatyana the following year and they remained together for the next decade.

War propelled Bulgakov into active medical service and he was drafted, still officially a student, to treat the wounded in a hospital in Saratov. Finally, in 1916, he was awarded a medical diploma and sent to work in a small country hospital in the depths of the Russian countryside. A single-handed practice, as it happens, with Tatyana as his nurse.

Bulgakov wrote up his experiences in this remote hospital in a series of short stories which he subsequently collected and published as *A Country Doctor's Notebook*.

The experience of working alone, isolated, newly qualified and 32 miles from the nearest town is one which must resonate with many doctors. That feeling of 'being thrown in at the deep end' is familiar to all juniors, in whatever specialty, and we can empathise with the country doctor as he struggles to apply his limited training and experience to whatever happens to stagger through the door out of the wild Russian night. The situations are graphically portrayed, the descriptions vivid and the doctor's fear is palpable as things drift out of control. In 'Baptism by Rotation', a transverse lie is corrected by lamplight. The young doctor rushes off to his study, on the pretext of fetching a cigarette, while his nurse prepares the woman for a chloroform anaesthetic:

> *There it was – Döderlin's Operative Obstetrics. I began hastily to leaf through the glossy pages. '... version is always a dangerous operation for the mother ...'*
>
> *A cold shiver ran down my spine.*
>
> *'The chief danger is the possibility of a spontaneous rupture of the uterus ...'*
>
> *Spon-tan-e-ous ...*
>
> *'If in introducing his hand into the uterus the obstetrician encounters any hindrances to penetrating to the foot, whether from lack of space or as a result of a contraction of the uterine wall, he should refrain from further attempts to carry out the version ...'*
>
> *Good. Provided I am able, by some miracle, to recognise these 'hindrances' and I refrain from 'further attempts', what, might I ask, am I supposed to do with an anaesthetised woman from the village of Dultsevo?*

And, a little further on:

> *What if the husband of the woman from Dultsevo is left a widower? I wiped the sweat from my brow, rallied my strength and disregarded*

all the terrible things that could go wrong, trying only to remember the absolute essentials: what I had to do, where and how to put my hands. But as I ran my eye over the lines of black print, I kept encountering new horrors. They leaped out at me from the page …

****

… I abandoned the Döderlin and sank into an armchair, struggling to reduce my random thoughts to order. Then I glanced at my watch. Hell! I had already spent twenty minutes in my room and they were waiting for me.
  '… with every hour of delay …'
Hours are made up of minutes, and at times like this the minutes fly by at an insane speed. I threw Döderlin aside and ran back to the hospital.

Inexperience is not the only source of Bulgakov's despair; his horror at the backwardness of the peasant population is a consistent theme throughout the book and the writer sees himself as a lone voice of reason in a sea of ignorance. Many of the stories take place at night, in storms and blizzards, and Bulgakov's dim surgery lamp is a pinpoint of enlightenment in a frightening and elemental darkness. There is an intense longing for home and civilisation, a growing disquiet and frustration and in 'Morphine', a telling account of the writer's resultant opiate addiction which he eventually overcame with the help of Tatyana.

The bloody revolution of 1918 saw Bulgakov in active service as a doctor in the White army, an experience he capitalised on in his novel *The White Guard* and his play *Flight*. Following an aborted attempt to emigrate via the Black Sea he gave up medicine for good and in 1921 moved to Moscow determined to make it as a writer in the new Soviet Union.

But for the remaining 19 years of his life Bulgakov struggled to be heard. No one would publish his books. First in the firing line was his satirical novella *The Heart of a Dog*.

'An acerbic broadside about the present age, there can be absolutely no question of publishing it …' was the reply the author received in 1925 from the publishing house Neda. Perhaps this wasn't entirely surprising. *The Heart of a Dog*, drawing heavily on Bulgakov's medical background, tells the tale of a bizarre experiment in

which a dog receives the transplanted testicles and pituitary gland of a recently deceased man. It is a fierce parable of the Russian revolution and the blackest of black comedies.

The following year the authorities closed down the journal *Rossiya* for serialising *The White Guard*. Bulgakov became targeted in the press as anti-Soviet, was blocked from publication or performance at every turn and his letters to the authorities are those of a man desperate to be freed.

Following an impassioned plea to the Central Committee in April 1930, Stalin, in a typical cat and mouse manoeuvre, phoned Bulgakov at home. One can only imagine the horrifying effect of such a call. Stalin asked the writer if he really wanted to leave the Soviet Union and if not, where would he like to work. Within four weeks Bulgakov had been appointed Assistant Director of the Moscow Arts Theatre, a post he held until his death in 1940. Bulgakov's experiences at the theatre are sardonically portrayed in his novel *Black Snow* and in the event were no less frustrating than those of the previous five years as a freelance author.

Throughout this miserable appointment, during which Bulgakov's plays were either banned or withdrawn from production, the writer was at work, in the evenings, throughout the night, but always in complete secrecy, on what was to prove his literary masterpiece, *The Master and Margarita*.

It is difficult to describe this extraordinary book, so kaleidoscopic is it, and so fantastically allegorical. In its style, *The Master and Margarita* prepares the ground for the magical realism of Gabriel Garcia Marquez and Milan Kundera, but it is more than an ephemeral fantasy. *The Master* is grotesque, a Faustian comic satire on a grand scale.

Professor Woland, a black magician, arrives in Moscow, ostensibly to put on a show, together with his two assistants: one seven feet tall but narrow in the shoulders, incredibly thin and with a face made for derision; the other, a large black cat capable of the most surprising acts.

[The cat] crouched, then leaped like a panther straight for Bengalsky's chest and from there to his head. Growling, the cat dug its claws into the compère's glossy hair and with a wild screech it twisted the head clean off the neck in two turns.

As Woland and his accomplices work their way through town, Moscow is soon in chaos as the vanity, greed and hypocrisy of its citizens is cruelly exposed. The hero of the book is a poet, the Master. Margarita is the woman he loves. We meet him first as an anonymous writer in a secure psychiatric clinic:

'I no longer have a name' replied the curious visitor with grim contempt. 'I have renounced it, as I have renounced life itself. Let us forget it.'

But amidst the ensuing madness, the Master's love and artistic integrity survives and he and Margarita finally, through death, achieve an everlasting peace. The idea of redemption through love pervades the book and interleaved throughout is a retelling, a most profound and sensitive retelling, of the final encounter between Christ and Pontius Pilate.

Regrettably it was not until 1973 that *The Master and Margarita* appeared unabridged for the first time. Since then, appreciation of the achievement that this novel represents has steadily grown and now, 60 years on, in a freer and more humane society, it assumes its rightful place as one of the classics of twentieth-century Western literature.

In a way, *A Country Doctor's Notebook* and *The Master and Margarita* are the bookends of Bulgakov's career. The former is an uncomplicated account of the challenges facing a youthful physician. The latter is a complex summing up of Bulgakov's own life, portraying the artist's relationship with an arbitrarily oppressive State and the ultimate triumph of love and art. Both portray the author as a lone figure battling against dark elemental forces. It is perhaps paradoxical that Bulgakov the doctor felt stifled by the superstitious stupidity of ordinary people, and felt himself unable to be understood. As a writer, he was systematically prevented from reaching out to that very proletariat by the people's representative, Josef Stalin – a Georgian peasant frightened of what luminous fires Bulgakov's creative spark might ignite.

Bulgakov's disillusionment with medicine, only exceeded by his disillusionment with artistic life in the Soviet Union, returned to dominate the last few months of his life. In 1939, the writer became ill from the hereditary renal disease that had killed his father. Fully aware of what was happening to him, and more importantly how powerless contemporary medicine was to do anything about it, Bulgakov became weak, emaciated and racked with pain. Bitter and exhausted, his acerbic wit did not desert him and shortly before he died, he wrote to his childhood friend Aleksander Gdeshinsky:

> I will add just one thing, towards the end of my life I have come to experience yet another disappointment – in therapeutic medicine. I won't call the doctors murderers, that would be too harsh, but I will willingly call them casual untalented hacks. There are exceptions of course, but they are rare!

The texts

A Country Doctor's Notebook, translation by Michael Glenny, was published by Collins and The Harvill Press in 1975.

The Master and Margarita was first published in serial form in Moskva (1966–67). An English translation by Richard Pevear and Larissa Volokhonsky was published by Penguin Books in 1997; translation by Michael Glenny published by The Harvill Press in 2000.

Further reading

Other novels by Bulgakov:

The White Guard (1991) The Harvill Press, London.

The Heart of a Dog (1989) The Harvill Press, London.

Biography:

Curtis J (1991) *Manuscripts Don't Burn, A Life in Letters and Diaries.* The Harvill Press, London.

14

Middlemarch

by George Eliot

Middlemarch has a special place in the affections of medical readers because it is a great novel which features a doctor as one of its central characters. Unfortunately for our professional pride, Dr Lydgate falls rather short of the mark as a hero, in spite of a promising start. Nevertheless, his story is a compelling one from which there is much to learn about how to be a doctor and how to be human. But our unfortunate colleague is not the only fascinating person you will meet when you read *Middlemarch*. It is a substantial novel of nearly 900 pages (don't be afraid), which interweaves a number of stories about people of different social status living in or near the fictitious Midlands town of Middlemarch in the early 1830s. Virginia Woolf famously called it 'one of the few English novels written for grown-up people'.

About the author

Perhaps I should begin by telling you a little about the author of this big book for grown-up readers. The first thing you need to know is that George Eliot was really a woman. She was originally called Mary Anne Evans but preferred when she was grown up to be called Marian. She was born in 1819, the daughter of a Warwickshire land agent. She was an earnest, serious little girl who wanted to be good and to do good in the world. She read only serious books and was eager to do helpful works about the parish. After the death of her mother when she was 16, her education began to broaden; she started to read more widely and became impressively well-informed; she fell in love several times but was generally disappointed – possibly her plain features and serious manner didn't appeal to the local boys. After a period as an evangelical Christian, she lost her religious faith without in any way giving up her moral purpose. She began to write articles for publication and, at the age of 32, landed a job as the editor of a journal called the *Westminster Review*. A few years later, we find her causing a scandal by 'eloping' and then setting up home with a married man, another writer called George Henry Lewes. Lewes encouraged her to write fiction and she soon became a great success. This was when she adopted the pen name of 'George Eliot'. The public loved her early novels such as *Adam Bede* and *The Mill on the Floss.* Queen Victoria was a great fan, although she couldn't meet Marian socially because she was still living in sin with George Henry. Their life together seems to have been a very happy one and Marian went on writing successful novels, some better than others. *Middlemarch*, which is definitely her best, was first published in 1870–71 in eight instalments, a new one appearing every two months. They must have been eagerly awaited, as readers would soon be hooked on the lives of the characters and be desperate to know what would happen next. And you will be, too; but you have the advantage of being able to possess the whole saga in one substantial volume.

Middlemarch: the story begins

Now it is time to open our shiny new copies of *Middlemarch* and plunge into the world that Marian has created for us. The book starts with a short prelude, which seems to be about St Theresa. If you find this puzzling (as I did) you can return to it later when it might make more sense. Book 1 (you remember there were eight instalments) is called 'Miss Brooke' and this is where we meet our principal heroine, a 19-year-old girl called Dorothea. Dorothea is a serious young woman (rather like the young Marian, but much prettier). She and her younger sister, Celia, have been adopted by their uncle, having lost their parents when they were 'about twelve'. Mr Brooke (as the uncle is always called) is a genial, well-meaning old fellow, a bit pompous, a bit tight-fisted, and definitely a silly ass, but you can't help liking him. The Brooke family are fairly upper class and they live in a posh estate called Tipton Grange, not far from Middlemarch, but in the country rather than the town. Social distinctions are important in Middlemarch society as we shortly see.

Now, sister Celia is a very open, sunny-natured girl, interested in boys rather than in books. But Dorothea is a bit of a puzzle, especially for the local young gentry. She is very good-looking and stands to come into plenty of wealth when her uncle dies. But she reads dusty old books on theology with great excitement and is full of schemes for improving the welfare of the farm workers. She has been known to kneel down in a humble cottage and pray with a sick labourer. Is that the sort of thing you want your wife to be doing? the men wonder; but she does look very sexy on horseback …

One young man, a neighbouring landowner and baronet called Sir James Chettam, decides that he will propose to Dorothea despite her imperfections. To everyone's surprise and dismay, Dorothea prefers another suitor, the reverend Mr Edward Casaubon, a clergyman and scholar, who at 45 is 'a dried up old bookworm'. He spends his time poring over ancient tomes and is known to be doing a great research project on the subject of mythology.

In Chapter 2, we are invited to a dinner party at which Mr Brooke and his nieces entertain both the red-whiskered young baronet (Sir James) and the distinguished middle-aged fossil. They talk of various subjects, including the application of science to agriculture and political economy. Mr Brooke's response in each case is that he has been there and done that already: 'I went into science myself a good deal at one time but I saw it would not do. It leads to everything; you can let nothing alone.' However, Dorothea makes some intelligent contributions and excites Mr Casaubon's interest. He notes that Dorothea is eager to sort out her uncle's papers and would clearly love to have her do the same for him.

Dorothea and Mr Casaubon

Later that evening when the two girls are alone, Celia says: 'How very ugly Mr Casaubon is!' Dorothea protests that he is one of the most distinguished-looking men she ever saw. She goes on to say that she believes he has a great soul. Poor Celia is dumbfounded. She loves and admires her big sister (for whom her pet name is Dodo) but she finds her very perplexing. Surely young James with his simple tastes and love of outdoor pursuits is the man to go for? Why would anyone want to marry a decrepit old buffer like Casaubon? But Dorothea is determined. When Sir James proposes, she turns him down. (He later turns to Celia instead and is happily accepted.) Now Mr Casaubon hands in a proposal to Dorothea in the form of a letter to her uncle. There is a touching and amusing scene in Chapter 4 when Mr Brooke tells Dorothea that Casaubon has asked for her hand and tries with great gentleness and kindness to persuade her not to say 'Yes'. 'He is over five-and-forty you know … To be sure, if you like learning and standing and that sort of thing, we can't have everything. And his income is good … Still he is not young, and I must not conceal from you my dear, that I think his health is not over-strong. I know nothing else against him.'

But Dodo is adamant. When she reads the letter she sobs with joy and gratitude. She is going to marry a distinguished scholar and she determines to dedicate her life to helping him in a humble capacity with his important researches. She even wonders if she is worthy of him. They meet and she talks to him for an hour 'pouring out her joy at the thought of devoting herself to him, and of learning how she might best share and further all his great ends'. Mr Casaubon (perhaps we should now call him Edward) kisses her brow and their fates are sealed.

Needless to say, this marriage shocks both family and friends. 'What business has an old bachelor like that to marry?' asks the aggrieved Sir James. 'He has one foot in the grave.' 'He means to draw it out again, I suppose,' observes the acidulous Mrs Cadwalladar, the rector's wife. We readers are a bit stunned as well and we wonder rather anxiously how this marriage is going to work out.

Not too well, I'm afraid. And there are early indications that both are due for a disappointment. Marian (George Eliot) gives us searching examinations of the minds of nearly all her characters. And when we look into Edward's mind we find him rather gloomily contemplating the fact that he doesn't feel the 'expected gladness' over his forthcoming union with a beautiful and passionate young girl. Is Marian trying to tell us in her Victorian way that the old boy is impotent? It seems very likely. And when they go on their honeymoon to Rome he doesn't even show any enthusiasm for seeing the sights, preferring her to go on her own while he buries himself in his research. When Dorothea tries to help him with his work, she gets another shock. He has stacks and stacks of notebooks but he hasn't even started writing his own book yet. And she discovers that he has failed to keep up with the latest work the Germans have been doing in his field (because he doesn't read German). In other words, as the scholars of our own age would no doubt put it, his research is crap. Marian's superb psychological observation makes this more poignant by letting us know that, deep down in his soul, Edward knows that as a scholar he is a failure. Dorothea is such a nice girl she would love to help and comfort him if only he would confide in her, but he is too scared. Her discomfort is made worse by an encounter in the Vatican with a young man called Will Ladislaw, who is actually a cousin of Edward's. Will is a real intellectual (he is the one who tips her off about the German literature) but he is also young, good-looking and full of the same kind of passionate feelings as our heroine. He is obviously her real soul mate – but she seems to have found him too late.

Enter Dr Lydgate

We are going to leave the Casaubons and their marriage for the moment because it is time to meet young Dr Lydgate, Middlemarch's newest general practitioner. Just before Dorothea's wedding, her uncle holds a dinner party at the Grange and graciously invites a few of the more distinguished members of the townsfolk of Middlemarch. The conversation turns (as so often it does) to illnesses and doctors. 'Tell me about this new surgeon, Mr Lydgate. I am told he is wonderfully clever,' says old Lady Chettam to the rector's wife. They agree that he is a gentleman, but Lady Chettam prefers a medical man to be 'more on a footing with the servants; they are often all the cleverer, I assure you. I found poor Hicks's judgement unfailing; I never knew him wrong. He was coarse and butcher-like, but he knew my constitution'. (That should be enough to put you off private practice.) Later on, we are allowed into the doctor's mind and we see Middlemarch from his point of view.

His first name is Tertius, but this is so preposterous that I am going to go on calling him Lydgate. He is just 27 and he has come to Middlemarch, like a newly qualified GP registrar, full of determination to be both a good doctor and a brilliant medical scientist. Oh really? Maybe we should take a look at his CV. He is a gentleman, yes, but he is not, strictly speaking, a physician. In those days, physicians were upper-class men who had been to Oxbridge and then became members of the Royal College of Physicians without ever learning much about the practicalities of treating patients. At a much lower social level were the apothecaries who hadn't been to the university and whose training was more of an apprenticeship. They were the predecessors of the modern general practitioner. But medical education was beginning to improve, especially in places like Edinburgh and Paris, where Lydgate has just completed his studies. Our boy is very confident and very ambitious. He means to make a name for himself as a medical scientist (he is very interested in something called 'the primitive tissue', which he believes must form the common histological basis of all the organs in the body); but he also wants to shine the bright clear light of evidence-based medicine on the dubious clinical practices of the older Middlemarch doctors. He is against old-fashioned and dangerous treatments such as bleeding and cupping; even more significantly, he wants to set an example to the others by refusing to dispense medicines himself. Furthermore, if there is no treatment known to be effective he would rather prescribe nothing. Now the other doctors are making a nice living by doing their own dispensing and filling their patients' stomachs with all sorts of expensive and unnecessary medicines. Not surprisingly, their reaction to Dr Lydgate is like that of your average PCG members when the clinical governance person sends round a circular: sceptical, derisory or downright hostile. As you can see, the medical scene hasn't changed that much in 170 years.

Lydgate also finds himself unwillingly involved in local politics when Middlemarch's prominent banker, Mr Bulstrode, offers to entrust him with the management of the new hospital he is financing. But he scores some striking successes with his patients, at least to begin with. His most significant patient is a young man called Fred Vincy, son of the mayor-elect of Middlemarch. Fred develops a headache and a fever after a day at the races and is soon very ill. The family's regular GP, Dr Wrench, visits once and sends some medicines but declines to visit again, dismissing Fred's illness as only 'a slight derangement'. In desperation, the family send for Lydgate, who suspects that Fred has typhoid fever. There were many fevers about in the 1830s and it was difficult to tell which was which, but typhoid was certainly one of them, and you may remember that headache is a significant early symptom. (Oh dear, and I promised myself never to teach medicine in these chapters.) Anyway, I am happy to say that Lydgate is very supportive, and young Fred makes a full recovery. We shall hear more of him later as he and his sweetheart Mary are the principals in the third narrative thread of *Middlemarch,* which our friend Marian is skilfully weaving.

Now, apart from the professional aspect, there is another reason why Dr Lydgate is very happy to visit Fred Vincy. Fred has a sister called Rosamond, who is very attractive. Lydgate enjoys a little flirtation with her but he reminds himself that he is definitely not even going to think about getting married until his career is more firmly established. But Rosamond has other ideas and she is used to getting what she wants. She likes Lydgate and she can tell that he is a proper gentleman, definitely a cut above the less-refined young men of lower-middle class Middlemarch. As the young people are frequently to be seen enjoying each other's company, the town begins to talk of an engagement; but no proposal is forthcoming from Dr Lydgate. Rosamond becomes quite distraught. Then one day, he stoops to picks up an ornamental chain that she has dropped and 'When he rose he was very near to a lovely little face set on a fair long neck.' Tears begin to cover her blue eyes and to fall over her cheeks and Lydgate is lost.

Well, you might say, why shouldn't they get married? They are obviously hot for each other, he seems to have good prospects and her Dad is going to be the mayor. They do get married, but soon there are big problems for these two innocents. Rosamond is proud of her husband but she is not particularly interested in medical research. She is much more interested in having expensive clothes and jewellery, good furniture and fine china in the house. Rosamond is not the sort of girl who can be trusted to be sensible with a credit card. She spends a serious amount of money and, as Lydgate's financial management isn't very good, they are soon deeply in debt, which Rosamond finds very humiliating. She is horrified when Lydgate says they will have to sell her jewels and auction the best furniture. And he is very angry when she secretly writes to his rich relatives in an unsuccessful plea for a loan. Even if Rosamond is a bit selfish, you can't help feeling sorry for both of them as things go financially from bad to worse. Despite these quarrels, he remains very devoted to her and their bedroom life is undoubtedly a lot better than that of Dorothea and her husband. It makes me wonder why Marian never thought of pairing Lydgate with Dorothea. Perhaps it is because the two stories were originally conceived separately and were very cleverly woven together. I will have more to say about Marian's writing skills later on.

Fred and Mary

Now it is time to look at a third pair of lovers. This time they are both ordinary townsfolk rather than landowners or professionals. We have already had a glimpse of Fred as Lydgate's patient, when he was suffering from typhoid, and you will remember that he is Rosamond's brother. Now Fred is the kind of amiable, good-natured young man who drives his parents mad with worry because he won't settle to anything and is constantly on the brink of going to the bad. He has been to university and he is supposed to be heading for a career in the church, although he clearly isn't suited to clerical life. He prefers hanging around in the billiard hall with his mates or trying to do clever horse deals in the nearby city. He gets into debt and hopes to inherit some money from his mother's old uncle, but his hopes in the end are dashed. (This is a good interpolated story which I haven't room to tell, but you'll find it in the book.) Fred's guardian angel is little Mary Garth, his childhood sweetheart. Mary's parents are also solid Middlemarch citizens. Her father, Caleb Garth, is a land agent and builder (rather like Marian Evans's father). Mary loves Fred dearly but she is very strict with him and makes it clear that she will never be his wife unless he starts to take life seriously and trains for a career. In a less monumental novel, Mary would do very well for a heroine, even though she is not at all glamorous. Marian gives a wonderful description of her in Chapter 40:

> *If you want to know more particularly how Mary looked, you will see a face like hers in a crowded street tomorrow ... fix your eyes on some small plump brownish person of firm but quiet carriage, who looks about her, but does not suppose anybody is looking at her ... she has a broad face, and square brow, well marked eyebrows and curly dark hair, a certain expression of amusement in her glance which her mouth keeps the secret of ... If you made her smile she would show you perfect little teeth; if you made her angry she would not raise her voice, but would probably say one of the bitterest things you have ever tasted the flavour of; if you did her a kindness, she would never forget it.*

I think that's just wonderful: a good illustration of Marian's writing at its best.

Mary's father, Caleb, is quite fond of Fred too and he offers to take him into the business. It is hard work and rather humbling (he has to learn to write in a good round clerical hand instead of an undergraduate scrawl and there is also a lot of manual work) but he gets down to it, gives up his juvenile ways, and is rewarded with Mary's unreserved and generous love. Theirs is the only story in the book which ends on an upbeat note. Some critics have observed that they and their families are content to carry on in the old pre-industrial revolution way of life, while the others (especially Dorothea and Lydgate) are eager for modernisation and social change. I don't think Marian was against progress – far from it – but she wants us to know that changing public opinion can be very hard work and your personal life may come to grief.

Bulstrode the banker

There is one more important character in *Middlemarch* whom we must meet because his actions have important consequences for many of the others. I have already mentioned that Dr Lydgate needs his patronage in order to be given a free hand to run the new hospital. Bulstrode has money, so naturally he is in a powerful position to give or withhold help to struggling Middlemarchers. He is a religious man and rather sanctimonious with it; but he has a very sympathetic wife who is Fred Vincy's father's sister. (There is a whole network of family connections in *Middlemarch* and, as so often in novel reading, it is well worth constructing a genogram as you go along.) Anyway, banker Bulstrode has a murky past which threatens to catch up with him when an old acquaintance turns up in the town and starts trying to blackmail him. Lydgate appeals to him for a loan to stave off his impending bankruptcy. At first Bulstrode refuses, but then he finds himself looking after the blackmailer who seems to be suffering from terminal alcoholism. Raffles (that is the man's name) has delirium tremens and becomes quite helpless. Lydgate is called in to supervise the treatment – and is surprised to find that Bulstrode is now quite eager to lend him money. Raffles very soon dies. Is Bulstrode responsible for his death? Did the doctor play a collusive role? People begin to talk again and suddenly Lydgate is out of favour. Patients are scared to call him in case he kills them with his modern experiments. According to Mrs Dollop, the landlady of The Tankard, 'There's been more going on than the prayer book's got a service for.' He and Rosamond have to leave town, and although they recover, it is the end of all his dreams of making a significant contribution to medicine. I did warn you that the poor fellow is not a doctor of heroic stature, set up for us to admire and emulate. But Marian does make us feel deeply for him and perhaps ponder a little about our own professional lives.

Portrait of a town

Another important 'character' in the book is the town of Middlemarch itself, portrayed at a time of transition from a rural to an industrial economy. As she relates her overlapping, interlocking stories, Marian takes us all over the town and the surrounding country, showing us the life of the community. We visit two pubs (The Green Dragon and the more downmarket Tankard) where all the gossip is exchanged and opinions are formed. We drop in on a furniture auction and take part in some dodgy horse-trading. We watch the first surveying of the land where the new railway will come thundering through, bringing the modern age with it, to the dismay and incomprehension of some of the farmers. We have dinner with some of the grander families and visit their estates. We sit in town meetings with the other worthy citizens. Most exciting of all, we get to take part in the 1832 general election, the first to extend the franchise in even a limited way to ordinary people. Mr Brooke, Dorothea's uncle, decides to stand as a Whig candidate, with Dorothea's soul mate, Will Ladislaw, acting as his spin doctor; I probably don't need to tell you that their campaign is a disaster but it is a very entertaining spectacle for readers and onlookers.

What happens to Dorothea?

At this stage you must be wondering if I have forgotten Dorothea. I have more or less told you how things work out for two of our couples, the Lydgates and Fred and Mary Vincy (as they will soon become). But I seem to have left Dorothea chained to the depressed and depressing Mr Casaubon. Well, I can reveal to you that her imprisonment does not last very long. As Mr Brooke foresaw, poor old Edward's health is not very good and it is not improved by a letter from his cousin Will Ladislaw. Will, you may remember is the young man who had such a powerful effect on Dorothea's feelings when they met on her honeymoon. Now Will has written to Dorothea to say he would like to come and visit – a proposal which her husband stiffly declines. (He has guessed that something is going on between these two, even if it only consists of silent passionate glances.) Dorothea flares up in anger (for the first time in their marriage), making Edward feel rather nervous. Half an hour later he has a typical attack of angina in the library. There is no mention of chest pain but he is gasping and 'seemed helpless and about to faint'. Dr Lydgate is called in and after listening to Edward's chest with the recently invented stetho-scope, he gives Dorothea a guarded prognosis. Her husband is advised to avoid 'stress and mental agitation'. Later on, he and Lydgate have a consultation as they walk together in the Yew Tree Walk. Lydgate tells him that he has 'fatty degeneration of the heart' and that he may die suddenly. Edward thanks him, politely, and we watch him walking off: 'a black figure with hands behind him and head bent forward continuing to pace the walk where the dark yew-trees gave him a mute companionship in melancholy, and the little shadows of bird or leaf that fleeted across the isles of sunlight stole along in silence as in the presence of a sorrow. Here was a man who now for the first time found himself looking into the eyes of death'. It is a wonderful description and there is more in that vein as the chapter continues. Dorothea has a last moment of tenderness and compassion for him. Then, a few days later, he asks her, if he dies, to promise 'to carry out my wishes'. What does he mean? Spend years trying to finish the research? She puts off giving him a straight yes or no; soon afterwards she finds him sitting alone in the summer house. He is very still and silent. He is dead.

Edward knew that Dorothea had been seeing quite a lot of Will and that there was a powerful chemistry between them. His 'wishes', embodied in his will, are that Dorothea does not marry Will and that if she does she will forfeit the inheritance of his property. But no matter; she has some money of her own, so there. After a terrific struggle to deal with his pride and her misplaced jealousy, I am happy to say that they do get married. I must also say (and I am not the first) that Will is a little disappointing as a husband for our Dorothea. He lacks solidity and vigour and doesn't really do anything brave and risky, although he is a decent enough chap, and heaven knows a great improvement on the unfortunate Edward. Marian wraps the story up in a short 'Finale', at the end of which she refers back to the prologue in which Dorothea is described as a sort of St Theresa who didn't quite make it. St Theresa was a woman of great zeal and energy who not only had mystic visions but founded and ran a religious order with great efficiency. In our day, she would have been the managing director of a major company. Dorothea has this potential but doesn't fulfil it, devoting herself instead to a life of quiet domesticity as Mrs Ladislaw. Nevertheless, Marian assures us, her goodness is 'incalculably diffusive' and has an influence on everyone she meets.

The author as therapist

Why doesn't our author allow her heroine to have her own career as a social reformer or perhaps a writer? After all, Marian herself defied social conventions and became a woman who was world famous for her own achievements rather than simply helping her husband. We don't really know. And yet, by the time we have finished reading her masterpiece we should know Marian pretty well. She is possibly the most important 'character' in the book. Although she does not have a part in the plot, her authorial presence is inescapable. While we observe the lives of her characters, she tells in detail what they are thinking and what makes them behave the way they do. She has compassion for everyone (although perhaps she is a little sharp with Rosamond at times) and reminds us that everyone is worthy of respect and attention. At one point (Chapter 29) she even catches herself being too partial and says: 'One morning … Dorothea, but why always Dorothea?' and takes instead on a journey to the interior of Casaubon's secret soul to remind us that he is also, in his strange way, human like the rest of us. Marian has a shrewd understanding of what makes all her characters' inner wheels revolve. She leans over your shoulder as you watch them, explaining why they feel and behave the way they do. I have to admit that I sometimes feel a sense of release when she gives us a few pages of straightforward storytelling; she is a bit like a wise psychotherapist whose interpretations are totally accurate, although not always what the client wants to hear. But that's the way George (Marian) Eliot is: you have to take the total package including the storyteller and the psychotherapist. After all, this is a story for grown-ups. So, when you feel you have had enough of *Harry Potter* for a while, why not give *Middlemarch* a try? You won't regret it.

The text

Middlemarch (1871–72) by George Eliot is available in Penguin Classics, with a good introduction by WJ Harvey.

15

If on a Winter's Night, a Traveller

by Italo Calvino

I love to read a straightforward story which draws me in from the beginning, makes me feel involved with all the characters, and promises me a long and enjoyable journey in congenial company until the book reaches its inevitable and satisfactory conclusion. They get married and they live happily ever after. But I also love books which are unruly and more than a bit unreliable; books whose authors tease you and have conversations with you and can't resist telling you: 'This story isn't really happening, you know; it's just something I've invented and I can change it any time I want to.' This may sound infuriating and indeed it often is – but if it's written by someone who is really gifted and full of charm you can forgive him all sorts of outrageous tricks because you want to see what he's going to do next. Does this remind you of anybody? If you have read *Tristram Shandy* (see Chapter 10) you might come to the conclusion that the tradition of the writer playing games with the reader began in the eighteenth century with Laurence Sterne.

My favourite twentieth-century literary trickster is the Italian novelist Italo Calvino (1923–1985), who has been very well translated into English by William Weaver. *If on a Winter's Night, a Traveller* is a funny title to begin with – it seems to break off in the middle of a sentence leaving you suspended uncomfortably on the end of a conditional clause. But when you open the book at Chapter 1, page 1, you find that the author has taken you firmly by the hand and is sitting you down to read his book! 'You are about to begin reading Italo Calvino's new novel, *If on a Winter's Night, a Traveller*, (he says). 'Relax. Concentrate. Dispel every other thought. Let the world around you fade.'

He goes on to advise you to close the door to the next room so you can't hear the TV and tell 'the others' to leave you in peace while you read. He follows with some advice about getting really comfortable, with a good light, having your cigarettes to hand, going to the loo if you have to and so forth. He then tells you the sort of person you are (which is a bit disconcerting, especially as he seems to get most of it right. Except perhaps the cigarettes). You are certainly a person who likes reading books so he then 'reminds' you how you went to the bookshop to buy your copy of *If on a Winter's Night*. There follows a wonderful riff about all the different sorts of books which you have to get past in the bookshop before you can purchase this one. They include Books You Needn't Read, Books You Mean To Read But There Are Others You Must Read First, Books You Can Borrow From Somebody and (my favourite) Books That Everyone's Read So It's As If You Have Read Them Too. Finally, you buy the book and Calvino describes how you get it home and unwrap it impatiently. He even describes you starting to read. And tells you that you can't recognise this author's 'unmistakable tone'. Come on, Italo, when is the real story starting? What are you trying to do to us? I suppose this might be called deconstructing the reading of a novel. He is certainly playing with us, his readers, and I can see that some people might find this pretty irritating, although as I've said, I really enjoy a bit of literary teasing. With a sigh of relief, we turn to Chapter 2 – actually it's not called Chapter 2, it's called 'If on a Winter's Night, a Traveller'. But we won't quibble, because at last the story appears to be starting! It appears to be a novel within the novel.

The novel begins in a railway station and it is beautifully written, a marvellously atmospheric invocation of a steamy, smoky, old station with a platform and a buffet – rather like the one in the film *Brief Encounter*. However, you can't help noticing that

Calvino is commenting on his literary technique all the time, almost as if he really was trying to describe a film. Gradually a plot emerges from the steam and smoke. The mysterious hero is some sort of secret agent trying to carry out a desperate mission involving a suitcase. He meets an attractive woman in the buffet and observes her relationship with her ex-husband, the doctor. The local police chief arrives and things begin to get exciting. The chief whispers to our unnamed hero: 'They've killed Jan. Clear out … catch the eleven o'clock express … you have three minutes.' Now it has become more like a Hitchcock film or a Graham Greene thriller. You turn the page eagerly to the next chapter – and find you have fallen into a trap! This is the real Chapter 2 and the author is addressing the reader directly again. He tells you (outrageously) that you find you are reading the same pages over again and in fact the book has been bound wrongly – all the rest of the pages are simply repeats of what you have read so far! (Be assured, this is not actually the case in the book you are reading, only in the book you think you are reading.) The best thing to do is to take the book back to the store and demand another copy. So this is what you do. You are given another copy: but it turns out to be a completely different story (with a different title). Does this sound complicated? It gets worse, so if you really don't like this sort of game I would advise you to get off here.

For those of you who are still with me (this kind of self-referential writing style is a bit infectious; I seem to be doing it too), I will stop following all the convolutions of this little master-piece and give you an idea of the overall structure of the book. The way it works (I think) is that there is an 'outer story,' which is all about reading books and the struggles of people who are trying to get hold of the books they desperately want. It is a story which starts in a bookshop and gradually takes you all over the world, getting progressively more fantastic and dangerous. I say 'dangerous' because 'you', the reader, are the hero of this outer tale whether you like it or not. You find yourself tangling with deceitful publishers, misleading translators, determined censors and even fanatical dictators in countries where books are regarded as dangerous and subversive. But it is not all bad. By way of compensation you are given a love interest in the shape of the 'other reader' (of the opposite gender) who shares your love of books and your determination to finish the one you are trying to read.

But there is a problem. It proves impossible to finish the story 'If on a Winter's Night, a Traveller' or indeed any other story in this maddeningly brilliant book. Oh yes, there are plenty of other stories. They make up the inner parts of the book. You see, each numbered chapter (of which there are 11 plus a little epilogue) in the outer tale is followed by the first chapter of a different inner 'novel'. None of these fictions is allowed to get past the first chapter and this could lead to a feeling of frustration and *lexus interruptus*. Not so with Calvino. Because, once you realise that they consist of only one chapter, each of these 'beginnings' is a perfectly composed short story, every one in a different style. Some have exciting cliffhanger endings (deliciously tantalising), while others land quite softly. They all conjure up different literary land-scapes: South American magical realist, North American thriller, East European political, Kafkaesque nightmare, Japanese erotic. All together they make up a wonderfully varied bunch of short stories – wrapped up in the 'outer story' of which you, the readers, are 'hero' and 'heroine.' And I don't think I'm giving away too much of a secret if I tell you that Calvino proves in the end to be quite a benign old-fashioned storyteller: on the last page you and the 'other reader' get married. In the last scene, you are in bed together and she says: 'Turn off your light, too. Aren't you tired of reading?' And you say, 'Just a moment. I've almost finished *If on a Winter's Night, a Traveller* by Italo Calvino.'

Afterthought

I have to admit that there are no wonderfully heart-warming characters in *If on a Winter's Night*. Its true subject is the joy of reading and that is one reason why I have included it, as well as its playfulness. It also occurs to me that the way the little stories keep breaking off and leaving you wondering – although it can be a touch frustrating – reminds me of something else. It is rather like the experience of doing a morning surgery. Someone whom you may never have seen before walks in and begins to tell you a story, which breaks off without reaching a conclusion. He or she is rapidly followed by another person with an entirely different story, which breaks off in its turn. Perhaps it will be continued another day. Perhaps not. And so it goes on until the surgery ends leaving you feeling slightly giddy and reaching gratefully for the cup of coffee cooling beside the sphygmomanometer.

The text

If on a Winter's Night, a Traveller by Italo Calvino was first published in 1979. The English translation by William Weaver (1981) is available in Harvest edition, Harcourt Brace and Company.

16

Bleak House

by Charles Dickens

How long is it since we actually read a novel by Dickens? His more colourful characters, like Mr Pickwick, Oliver Twist and Ebenezer Scrooge are so well known to us that they seem to lead an existence quite independent of the books. Then there are the films, the musicals, the cartoon strips. We seem to know all about Dickens. His world is already so familiar that we wonder if we really need to read the books. After all, they are quite formidable-looking when we run an eye along a shelf full of them. But once we have prised one out and taken it away with us, we are in for a special treat of the kind which only reading can provide. But which one to choose? I could have gone for a straightforward bio-graphical story like *David Copperfield* or *Great Expectations*. Instead, some powerful force led me back to a strange, murky, very mysteri-ous, very atmospheric Dickens masterpiece called *Bleak House*. The very name can induce a chill feeling down the spine. But what is it about and what do its 900 pages and 67 chapters have waiting for us?

Dickens wrote it when he was about 40 and published it initially in 20 monthly parts (1852–53) before it appeared in a single volume in 1853. It has a complex plot (which will in due course be laid before you) and a generous helping of larger-than-life Dickensian characters. Some are colourful and lovable, some are grotesque and bizarre and many are decidedly creepy. There are some pathetic little children, a totally benign middle-aged gentleman and several people you would take care to avoid at parties. You will be glad to hear that there is a little orphan heroine who is not only sweet and good-natured but plucky and determined. You will sigh contentedly when she finds true happiness at the end of the book. This is all exactly as it should be in a Dickens novel.

But perhaps the most important 'character' in the book is the early Victorian City of London described exactly as it was – or perhaps not quite as it was but modulated by the feelings and imagination of the amazing Charles Dickens. That you must decide for yourselves, because it's time to get started.

Bleak House: the story begins ...

The story really has three beginnings, represented by the first three chapters. Chapter 1 is one of the best Dickens ever wrote. Using brown, muddy, foggy colours he paints a vivid word picture of a foggy, muddy, filthy, wintry London. Everyone who writes about *Bleak House* quotes from the opening and who am I to resist it? Here we go ...

> LONDON. Michaelmas Term lately over, and the Lord Chancellor sitting in Lincoln's Inn Hall. Implacable November weather. As much mud in the streets as if the waters had but newly retired from the face of the earth and it would not be wonderful to meet a Megalosaurus, forty feet long or so, waddling like an elephantine lizard up Holborn Hill. Smoke lowering down from chimney pots, making a soft black drizzle, with flakes of soot in it as big as full-grown snow flakes – gone into mourning, one might imagine, for the death of the sun. Dogs, indistinguishable in mire. Horses, scarcely better; splashed to the very blinkers. Foot passengers, jostling one another's umbrellas, in a general infection of ill-temper, and losing their footing at street corners ...

That's the mud and the soot; now here comes the fog:

> Fog everywhere. Fog up the river, where it flows among green aits and meadows; fog down the river, where it rolls defiled among the tiers of shipping, and the waterside pollutions of a great and dirty city. Fog on the Essex marshes, fog on the Kentish heights.

I'll skip a bit here but you can read it all, and we come to: 'Gas looming through the fog.' What a phrase! I guess he means gas light because:

> Most of the shops lighted two hours before their time – as the gas seems to know for it has a haggard and unwilling look. The raw afternoon is rawest and the dense fog is densest and the muddy streets are muddiest near that leaden headed obstruction ... Temple Bar. And hard by Temple Bar, in Lincoln's Inn Hall, at the very heart of the fog, sits the Lord High Chancellor in his High Court of Chancery.

Dickens has led us through the mud and the fog to the courtroom, where the legal and intellectual fog is more than a match for the murk and gloom outside. He goes on to give us a brilliant satirical sketch of the lawyers and their unfortunate clients in this most obscure of courts. (I wish I could quote the whole chapter, but I must restrain myself, and you absolutely must read it for yourselves, over and over again with relish.) What is the case which the Lord Chancellor is hearing? The case of Jarndyce and Jarndyce, an incredibly tortuous and long drawn out dispute about a will in the Jarndyce family which has been running for years without any sign of coming to a conclusion. This is great sport for the lawyers but wretched for the clients because Dickens makes it clear to us that any money they might hope to be awarded will all be swallowed up in costs. As we sit in court, peering through the fog at the scarlet-robed Lord Chancellor and the bobbing, bowing, droning barristers, we become aware of some of the victims of Jarndyce and Jarndyce who are caught up in the terrible business. There is 'a little mad old woman in a squeezed bonnet' (we shall meet her later); another poor wretch who keeps being sent back to prison for contempt of court because he is so enraged by it all; and 'the man from Shropshire' who keeps trying (without success) to attract the Lord Chancellor's attention with sonorous shouts of 'My lord!' (He is a bit like the patient who tries to attract your attention as you sweep through the waiting room on an urgent mission to get a cup of coffee.)

Chapter 2 transports us to the London house of Sir Leicester and Lady Dedlock. The Dedlocks' country seat is a house called Chesney Wold in Lincolnshire (which we shall also be visiting).

But just now, the Dedlocks have retreated to town because in Dickens' Lincolnshire there is perpetual rain, 'and the heavy drops fall drip, drip, drip upon the broad flagged pavement called, from old time, The Ghost's Walk, all night.'

Sir Leicester is an elderly baronet, probably, Dickens estimates, in his late sixties, very stiff and respectable. His lady is 20 years younger and, while she is still beautiful, her glacial demeanour tells us that she has been pretty seriously damaged by some suffering or other. When we arrive to spy on them, the Dedlocks are talking to their family solicitor, an old gentleman called Mr Tulkinghorn, who is so old-fashioned he wears knee breeches (which were out of date even then). You won't be surprised to hear that the Dedlocks have an interest in the case of Jarndyce and Jarndyce and Mr Tulkinghorn has come to give them an update on its progress (going nowhere, naturally.) But the arresting, heart-stopping moment in this chapter comes when old Tulkinghorn shows Lady Dedlock a document which has been copied by a legal clerk whose handwriting she seems to recognise. She goes very pale, almost faints and has to be taken to her room. '"I never knew my lady swoon before," murmurs Sir Leicester. "But the weather is extremely trying – and she really has been bored to death down at our place in Lincolnshire."'

Esther takes over

What a way to end a chapter. And what on earth is going on? We turn the page to Chapter 3 and find yet another new beginning. This time the story is being told in a new voice, that of a young woman who has slipped her small hand into ours and is telling us her life story. The young woman is Esther Summerson, the heroine of *Bleak House* and from now on she will be responsible for nearly half of the chapters. She begins with characteristic modesty: 'I shall have great difficulty in beginning to write my portion of these pages, for I know I am not very clever.'

Esther tells us about her solitary, orphan childhood in the care of her godmother with only her faithful Dolly to confide in. On her 13th birthday her godmother tells her that it would have been better if she had never been born: 'Your mother, Esther, is your disgrace and you were hers.' Shortly afterwards, the godmother dies and Esther finds herself placed under the care of a mysterious guardian who arranges for her to go to school and get a decent education. Six years pass quite happily until, at the age of 20, young Esther is summoned to London to live in her guardian's house as a companion for his new ward. Her guardian's name is Mr John Jarndyce, so we immediately spot a connection with the notorious lawsuit described in Chapter 1. But Mr John is as benign a gentleman as you could hope to meet in a Dickens novel and, although his father was driven to suicide by the lawsuit, he himself has sensibly decided to have nothing to do with it. He does, however, in his generosity, act as guardian to two young cousins, Richard and Ada, who are also part of the Jarndyce family. And Esther has been brought in to act as companion for Ada. It is a bit difficult to understand where these two have sprung from, but never mind, they are very friendly to Esther, even if she is somewhat below them in social status. We even get to meet the Lord Chancellor in his private rooms in this chapter as he has to give his consent to the wardship arrangements. Outside his office the three young people have their first meeting with the bird-like little woman called Miss Flite who has been hoping for a favourable outcome from the Jarndyce case.

> "Mad!" whispered Richard, not thinking she could hear him.
> "Right! Mad, young gentleman," she returned so quickly that he was quite abashed. "I was a ward myself, once. I was not mad at the time," curtseying low and smiling between every little sentence. "I had youth, and hope. I believe, beauty. It matters very little now. Neither of the three served or saved me. I have the honour to attend court regularly. With my documents. I expect a judgment. Shortly. On the day of Judgment."

More weird Dickensian characters

Richard has an ominous connection with Miss Flite, because preoccupation with the case is destined to drive him to the brink of insanity as well. But that lies a long way in the future. And we have lots more Dickensian characters to meet. There are so many that I shall have to leave you to interview some of them by yourselves or else I shall lose the plot entirely. The next chapter (4) introduces the Jellyby family. Mrs Jellyby is a philanthropist who spends so much of her time and energy on trying to set up projects in Africa to improve the lot of the natives, that she grievously neglects to look after her own children, who are ill-fed, unwashed, poorly clothed and constantly having accidents. I suppose the modern equivalent might be a workaholic doctor who never has any time or thought for his own family. So look on Mrs Jellyby and be warned.

Our good-natured Esther befriends the Jellyby children, especially the elder daughter, Caddy, who is used by her mother as a secretarial drudge. Caddy and Esther go for a walk on a foggy London morning and Dickens carefully guides them (and us) towards the courts and alleys surrounding Lincoln's Inn. Here they again come across little Miss Flite who invites them into her lodgings. She rents a room over a weird junk shop full of ancient legal bric-a-brac and owned by Mr Krook, a sinister old man 'short, cadaverous and withered'. Krook is known as the Lord Chancellor, because the heap of dusty legal rubbish over which he presides is a sort of ghastly mockery of the court of Chancery itself. Krook treats the young people to a grisly account of how old Tom Jarndyce was driven to despair and suicide by the interminable process of the court. He seems to find it all highly amusing. I should also tell you that Krook has a large grey cat called Lady Jane, who is perhaps the most horribly evil cat in English fiction. And I speak as a cat lover.

In her room above the shop, Miss Flite keeps a large number of songbirds in cages. She intends to give them their freedom on the 'day of judgement' when the case is concluded, in her favour, as she hopes and believes. But that cat, Lady Jane, stalks round eyeing them hungrily. One feels that she will pick them clean just as the law in the real court of Chancery will demolish the hapless suitors. It's a very creepy thought and it makes me shiver. Dickens is such a brilliant writer. Who cares if he gets a bit sentimental over heroines like Esther? Now where was I? Oh yes, in Krook's legal rag-and-bottle shop. The shop is full of old parchments and papers, but Krook himself cannot read or write, although he is able to copy letters and chalk them on the walls. Krook will, in time, die a very strange death, which will send you back to your textbooks to see if it could possibly be true.

Bleak House: 'Quite at home'

Let us now follow the young people (Esther and her new friends, Ada and Richard) away from London and into the Hertfordshire countryside to the home of their guardian and patron, the benevolent Mr Jarndyce. The house is a pleasant rambling one and although it is called 'Bleak House' in memory of the suicidal Tom, it is to become a very cheerful home for the three young people. John Jarndyce is nearly always in a good mood, except when the suffering of a fellow creature begins to distress him. Then he retreats to a special study called the Growlery where he can growl in peace and decide what to do. Mr Jarndyce hands Esther the keys of the house, thus doing her the honour of making her his trusted housekeeper and at the same time reminding us that her status is a little below that of the two wards.

Comfortably installed in one of the sitting rooms we find an old friend of Mr Jarndyce called Harold Skimpole (another famous Dickens character). I must tell you a bit about Skimpole. At first, he seems rather attractive but, as his character is revealed, we find him more and more disturbing. Although middle-aged, he tells us blithely that he is a mere child. He is incapable of taking any responsibility and lives simply to enjoy himself. He knows nothing about money and prefers not to talk about it, but he is always happy to accept money and very adept at getting his indulgent friends to part with it. Is Harold a charming innocent whose frankness is beguiling and his company delightful as he prattles away wittily? Or is he a rather callous, self-serving sponger? You must decide for yourselves. He is certainly at his most winning in this chapter as he fends off a bailiff who has come to arrest him for debt. I should tell you that Mr Skimpole has a degree in medicine – but he had to give up his one and only post as personal physician to a German prince because, when his services were required 'he was generally found lying on his back in bed, reading the newspapers, or making fancy-sketches in pencil, and couldn't come'.

So he is not one of our more admirable literary doctors, but Dickens has another one up his sleeve who will more than compensate: the wonderful, idealistic GP Dr Woodcourt, who is just the sort of young man we hope and expect will produce some palpitations in young Esther's girlish heart. But that meeting lies some way ahead.

The shock of poverty

Our next excursion takes us to meet some of Esther's neighbours in her new home. Dickens takes this opportunity to introduce some more of his hypocritical, middle-class, social do-gooders. Prominent among these is Mrs Pardiggle, who loves getting people to take out regular subscriptions to her good causes, even making her children part with their pocket money to set an example. She also likes visiting the poor in order to urge them to wash more often and to read the improving little books she leaves for them. (Since they don't know how to read this is rather pointless.) Esther is taken along to visit a poor brickmaker's family and Dickens seizes his chance to show us what the lives of the very poor were really like. How did he know? He had got into the habit ever since his adolescence of wandering around obscure and probably dangerous London slums, observing people and listening to them. The brickmaker's young wife has a black eye (a blow from her violent husband) and a baby on her lap. As we watch them, the baby dies. This is truly shocking and brings us up with a lurch. In the middle of the gentle satire on ridiculous people, we are given a sudden dose of brutal early-nineteenth-century reality. Esther does her best to help comfort the mother and her friends – and she begins to grow up a little more. In the next chapter, she receives a proposal of marriage from an earnest (but rather devious) young lawyer's clerk called William Guppy. Mr Guppy says he might be able to 'advance her interests' by way of ferreting out some evidence. What is he talking about? It is not yet clear. But Guppy is one of a whole crowd of characters in *Bleak House* who are searching for bits of paper, letters and documents bearing a certain handwriting – which they feel sure will lead to financial gain. Some of them can't even read, but this makes them even more eager to find the bits of writing. What is it all about? We shall have to wait a bit to find out because *Bleak House* is a mystery story among many other things. But you may well get some clues from the next chapter (10).

Death of a law writer

Now we are back in London, in Cook's Court, Cursitor Street, off Chancery Lane, in the heart of the legal district. If you go there today you will find that it is called 'Took's Court' and the old house at number 14 is a barristers' chambers headed by Michael Mansfield QC. Our business is with Mr Snagsby, who is a law stationer: that is, he provides all the bits and pieces that lawyers need for writing – parchment, paper, pens, ink, sealing wax, rulers. Yes, the obsession with writing continues. Mr Snagsby lives with his fearsome wife and their servant Augusta (known as Guster), who is a poor drudge of a girl with no life of her own and, of course, no chance of an education despite being surrounded with pens and paper. Along to Mr Snagsby's comes old Mr Tulkinghorn, Sir Leicester Dedlock's lawyer, who lives just around the corner. He is clutching the document with the handwriting which caused Lady Dedlock to go pale and nearly faint in Chapter 2. (Turn back and read it again if you don't remember.) It seems that a lot of legal documents have to be reproduced (there being no photocopiers or laser printers) and part of Mr Snagsby's job is to 'give out' the work to poor scriveners trying to earn a living by doing handwritten copies.

Shrewd old Tulkinghorn has guessed that Lady Dedlock recognised the handwriting on this particular document and if she fainted it must have been that of someone who meant a lot to her. Clearly it is not that of her husband and Mr T means to find out who it was. Snagsby says the work was done by a fellow called 'Nemo', which the educated lawyer knows is Latin for 'no one'. But who is Mr Nobody? They rush over to his lodgings, which just happen to be in Krook's rag-and-bottle shop by Lincoln's Inn Fields. Mr Krook lights a candle and takes them up to the clerk's shabby little room (this is really creepy and exciting). Nemo is lying on his bed, a ragged, unshaven figure. The air in the room smells bad; 'but through the general sickliness and faintness, and the odour of stale tobacco, there comes to the lawyer's mouth the bitter, vapid taste of opium'. The unknown copyist is dead. (That's two deaths already: the total will be nine before we have finished.)

A witness at the inquest

Death is certified by a young surgeon, Allan Woodcourt (who has not yet encountered our Esther, who will become the love of his life). Since there has been a death in suspicious circumstances, there must be an inquest. This is held, by the custom of the time, in the local pub, The Sol's Arms. The coroner discovers that the deceased has only ever been seen to speak to one person – and that was 'the boy that sweeps the crossing down the lane over the way round the corner'. Yes, it is Jo, the crossing sweeper, one of Dickens' most important child poverty victims. Because he has absolutely nothing and no hope of anything he has been seen as the very bottom of the towering, tottering, rotting social order which Dickens reveals to us in *Bleak House*.

So let's meet little Jo. 'Here he is, very muddy, very hoarse, very ragged … Name, Jo. Nothing else that he knows on. Don't know that everybody has two names. Never heerd of sich a think. Don't know that Jo is short for a longer name. Thinks it long enough for *him*. – *He* don't find no fault with it. Spell it? No. *He* can't spell it. No father, no mother no friends. Never been to school.' But he does remember the dead man (with his yellow face and black hair). The man would ask him how he was and, when he had any, give him some money. '"He was wery good to me," says the boy, wiping his eyes with his wretched sleeve.'

Little Jo (we are never told exactly how old he is) lives in a hellish slum called Tom-All-Alone's; it is a heap of overcrowded, filthy, decaying tenements, where the rain easily penetrates and infectious fevers are a constant companion. Every so often, one of the rickety houses collapses with a crash and a cloud of dust. In this dismal place, shortly after the inquest, Jo receives a visit from a veiled lady who wants to know if he was the boy who was examined at the inquest. She then asks Jo to show her all the places connected with the deceased law writer, including where he lived and the graveyard where he was buried. He can see that, behind her veil she is deeply affected, especially by the pitiful, anonymous little common burial plot, screened by an iron gate. '"There," says Jo, pointing. "Over yinder, among them piles of bones …".'

Dickens takes care that we shall identify the mysterious lady without too much difficulty, despite her disguise. It is, of course, Lady Dedlock, on the trail of the author of the handwriting which had such a devastating effect on her in Chapter 2. But what is he to her and she to him? And what does all this have to do with young Esther and the lawsuit in Chancery and the fog and the mud and little Jo? Be assured that we shall find out, but not just yet.

A pause to take stock and consider

I have now introduced you to most of the important characters in *Bleak House* and we have travelled together through the first dozen or so chapters. By this time I hope that any misgivings you may have had about tackling a large work by Dickens will have vanished and you will be eager to get started. You no longer need my services as a personal escort on the rest of the journey. Besides, I am conscious of the fact that if I go on in my present fashion I shall end up writing a work of Dickensian proportions myself. Already my style is beginning to imitate the master's mixture of grand ironic rhetoric and gritty social reportage. So, from now on I shall not be with you every step of the way. Instead I shall be hovering above you, summarising the main themes, signposting the main twists of the plot and providing a synopsis of the further adventures of the main characters (while bringing in a few new ones).

Plots, characters and theme

Jarndyce and Jarndyce

The first plot we come across (Chapter 1) is the apparently endless story of the law suit of Jarndyce and Jarndyce as it grinds its way through the court of Chancery. The legal process may seem just stupid and boring, but we realise that because it feeds on human greed and addiction, it is also very destructive. Its victims include not only Miss Flite (and her birds, remember to look for their names, they have wonderful names), but Esther's young friends Richard and Ada, 'the wards in Jarndyce'. These two fall in love and become engaged. But Richard becomes obsessed with the case, from which he hopes to inherit a fortune and fails to train for a steady profession (he tries both medicine and the law). In the end, surprisingly, the case does finish. Unsurprisingly, only the lawyers benefit.

The paper chase

We have already observed that a sample of a dead man's handwriting on a legal document has provoked the intense interest of Mr Tulkinghorn, the Dedlock family lawyer, and induced Lady Dedlock herself to go wandering desperately around the slums of London in search of a ragged boy who might have some information. But other people are interested too. There is Mr Guppy (the legal clerk who proposed to Esther) and his rather sad friend Tony Jobling. And they have a friend called Smallweed, who is the grandson of a pair of elderly Smallweeds, gnarled, shrunken, grasping characters, who are indecently eager to get their hands on another sample of the same writing. This is in the form of a letter, in the possession of an old friend of the writer whose name, by the way, was Captain Hawdon. Yes, the deceased law writer was an ex-military man who wrote a letter to another retired soldier, a rather upright and honest chap called George, who keeps a shooting gallery. Guppy and Jobling are also on the trail of some more of the dead man's private papers which they believe to be in the possession of old Krook, the rag-and-bottle man. (Remember him? The one with the cat.) Of course, old Krook can't read, so how does he know *what* papers he has got hold of until someone sees them and deciphers them? Krook agrees to show his papers to the two young men and arranges to meet them at midnight one evening in his house (Chapter 32). This is a very strange chapter. It is creepy to start with because Tony Jobling is living in the very room where Captain Sawdon, the law writer, perished from an overdose of opium. As the two young men wait for 'the appointed time' they become aware of horrible burning smells, thick yellow liquid dripping from a windowsill and an even greater number than usual of sooty flakes in the air. When they reach Mr Krook's parlour downstairs they find that Krook and his bundle of letters have been reduced to a little pile of ashes and a burnt patch on the floor. Ladies and gentlemen, Mr Krook has undergone spontaneous combustion. Do you believe that's possible? Dickens did and insisted on its scientific status in his preface. And when you read this you will almost believe it too.

Hastily removing ourselves from the obscene sights and smells of Krook's shop (take care of that cat which is still crouching there and snarling), we might wonder why so many people want to get hold of these letters. Obviously money has something to do with it. If Lady Dedlock had a secret lover (which is possible, isn't it?), then she or Sir Leicester could be blackmailed. And that would explain why Mr Tulkinghorn in his role as family *consigliore* is anxious to prevent their getting into the wrong hands.

The murder mystery

I must apologise, because I have not had time, until now, even to hint that there is a murder mystery in *Bleak House*. My only excuse is that the assassination is committed fairly late in the book. The victim is old Mr Tulkinghorn, whom we follow home to his house one night only to find him lying dead under the pointing finger of a Roman soldier who is part of a painting on the ceiling of his sitting room. This is a gripping chapter illustrated by one of the wonderful pictures provided for Dickens by Hablot K Browne (better known as 'Phiz'). When you have a murder you must also have a detective and Dickens gives us one of the earliest portraits of a professional sleuth in English literature. His name is Inspector Bucket 'of the detective' (the Metropolitan Police had just started a CID branch of that name, so this was very topical, and Dickens had befriended and eulogised Inspector Field). Don't be deceived by Inspector Bucket's faintly ludicrous name: he is a very shrewd and tough cop indeed, although he does make mistakes. I will leave you to read and enjoy the various false clues and one false arrest (part of Bucket's plan) which lead eventually to the apprehension of the killer.

Lady Dedlock's story

Lady Dedlock remains a rather distant and chilly figure for most of the book; but she does acquire some pathos towards the end and we find ourselves warming to her a little more as her plot unfolds. The paper chase enthusiasts are constantly on her track looking for proof of her long-ago secret love affair with Captain Hawdon, the deceased law writer. Mr Tulkinghorn (as long as he lives) and Inspector Bucket try equally industriously to prevent the secret from coming out, but in order to protect the reputation of the Dedlock family rather than out of any kindness towards my lady. We have seen how Lady Dedlock rushes off into the lower depths of London to try and find the last traces of the life and death of the man she really loved. She does find some happiness when she discovers that the child they had is alive and well. They have a touching meeting with tears and embraces under a tree in the grounds of Chesney Wold. I don't think I shall be giving too much away when I tell you that my lady's long-lost daughter, born out of Dedlock, is none other than our young friend and narrator, Esther Summerson!

Esther's story

What has been happening to Esther since we left her, politely turning down Mr Guppy's proposal in the sitting room of Bleak House? Well, she continues (as she modestly tells us) to be as helpful as she can to all her friends and everybody she encounters. She looks after Bleak House for her guardian and is an ever-supportive counsellor to Ada and Richard. She helps the charitable Mrs Jellyby's elder daughter, Caddy, to escape from her oppressive home and marry her boyfriend. And she continues to embody Dickens' concern and compassion for the poor and dispossessed. I shall give you one important example. In Chapter 15, prompted by a careless remark of Mr Skimpole's that the man who tried to arrest him for debt has died leaving three orphan children, Esther's guardian, John Jarndyce, takes her off on another excursion into the slums. They find two children (Tom, 5, and Emma, one and a half) locked in their cold little room for safety while their big sister Charley (13) goes out to work scrubbing to support them. When Charley returns we are impressed and moved by her sense of responsibility for her little siblings. We are also relieved that she is not a child prostitute (although in reality she might well have been). Anyway, the little ones are provided for by benevolent Mr Jarndyce and Charley eventually becomes Esther's faithful maid and companion.

A further train of events (which I cannot describe in detail) will lead to poor Charley catching smallpox and being nursed by Esther, who then catches it too. She quarantines herself (to protect her dear Ada and the other residents of Bleak House), and is in turn nursed by Charley. She goes temporarily blind and her face becomes scarred permanently (no details, but she gives us to understand that she has lost whatever beauty she had). But at least she survives and recovers her strength. She escapes being sucked into the lawsuit like Richard and Ada; and she eventually meets and is (briefly) united with her mother, before that lady unhappily dies in her distraction.

But what about Esther's love life? She has various meetings with Allan Woodcourt, the young doctor, in which they clearly express an interest in each other. He disappears overseas for a large part of the book. Then we hear from Miss Flite that he has been doing heroic deeds rescuing people from a wrecked ship in '*the East India Seas*'. Esther's heart glows for her friend but she resigns herself to the fact that, since she has lost her beauty to the smallpox virus, there can be no possible hope of wedding bells. Well, I scarcely need to reassure you that a totally wonderful young physician like Allan Woodcourt is not going to be put off by a few pock marks on the face of such an angelic heroine as Esther. The wedding bells do indeed chime (after an alarming period when it seems she might be going to marry her guardian out of sheer altruism) and in the closing chapter we leave Esther in utter contentment in her new home in Yorkshire (called Bleak House, naturally) and her new life as the wife of a country doctor. Which is the perfect prescription for a happy life, I am sure you will agree. (Although Emma Bovary would raise a dissenting voice, see the next chapter.)

Dickens and the social system

This is not really a plot so much as a theme which underpins the structure of the novel. In the course of the book, we look at all the different layers of English society as Dickens saw them. At the top of the heap are the aristocrats like the Dedlocks, who are quite secure, at least for a while (except, as in Lady Dedlock's case, when their emotions overwhelm them). Society is controlled on their behalf by the political parties who, Dickens tells us, are identical and interchangeable for all the effect they have. He refers to their leaders as Lord Coodle and Sir Thomas Doodle. A little lower down are the middle classes, who include all the lawyers, scurrying around serving their masters and lining their own pockets. Also at this level are the 'philanthropists', for whom he reserves some of his bitterest satire, and the totally self-centred, comfortably off people like Harold Skimpole. There is only one character who has been able to pull himself up from his working-class origins and become a new age industrial 'ironmaster' creating employment for other people. This is Mr Rouncewell, the son of Sir Leicester's housekeeper who has some memorable confrontations with the master (for example, Chapter 22). At the bottom of the pyramid are the people in desperate poverty and especially the children for whom no one in the higher strata seems to care in the least. But Dickens cared. By the 1850s he was writing factual reports of the life of the poor and vigorously expressing his ideas in his journals *Household Words* and *All the Year Round*, and discussing strategy with practical social reformers such as Lady Burdett-Coutts. From his personal observations he knew that housing and education were important reforms on which money needed urgently to be spent. However, Alistair feels that dirt and disease were even more serious threats to Victorian city-dwellers, as he will tell us in his postscript.

In conclusion

That's all I have to say about *Bleak House*. I hope that you will go and read it and enjoy it as much as I have done. Some of the chapters are so amazingly written that you can read them over several times, letting them sink deeper into your soul. Some people complain that too many of his characters are either gross caricatures like Mr Krook, or sentimental idealisations like Mr John Jarndyce, Esther's ever-benevolent guardian. I must say that I don't find this a problem and I enjoy reading about all of them.

The text

Bleak House by Charles Dickens was first published in one volume in 1853. It is available in Penguin Classics with an introduction and helpful notes. I also found useful background material in *The World of Charles Dickens* by Angus Wilson, Penguin Books, 1970.

Postscript: 'Filthy Book' by Alistair Stead

Perhaps John's account does not do full justice to what I take to be a major impulse behind the writing of *Bleak House*, one seen now as freshly relevant to a society made so epidemiologically aware by, for instance, the menace of *E. coli*, mad cow disease and CJD, the inadequate hygiene of our hospitals. In publishing this novel in 1851–52, Dickens was not just writing opportunistically in a period when terrifying epidemics were sweeping through London (there were notable outbreaks of cholera in 1848 and 1854). Both from direct observation and from reading Edwin

Chadwick's critical Report on the Sanitary Conditions of the Labouring Population (which he had received from the brother-in-law who would go on to be appointed Chief Inspector for the Board of Health), he had become an informed and passionate campaigner for the indispensable proper sanitation of the metropolis and its environs. And, if his speech to the Metropolitan Sanitary Association in February 1850 was his most signal effort as the concerned citizen, his great – perhaps filthiest – novel may from time to time sound this note of declamatory zeal but, more often, finds subtler and more imaginative means of expounding and exploring the extent and menace of urban squalor.

What interconnects so many characters and incidents in the book is disease (then believed to be borne on 'fog and filthy air') and dirt. While the legal deadlock of Chancery, and the Jarndyce and Jarndyce case in particular, generally brings about mental instability and collapse, the very names of Chancery (cf cancer) and Jarndyce (cf jaundice) suggest contamination by the novel's equally, maybe substantially more, graphic preoccupation with threats to the physical wellbeing of most city-dwellers. Although the bravura opening to the story has a double-headed concern with mud and fog, symbolic of the interdependent social ills of a polluted environment and a mystifying, outdated legal system, I would ask you to pay more attention to that omnipresent mud, merely the first of innumerable variations on the theme of dirt – for which we may read, in many instances, the ordure which the Victorian novelist's literary decorum cannot name. In 1880, Ruskin, fulminating memorably, even crazily, against modern trends to morbidity in fiction, indicts *Bleak House* for its accumulation of (often sensational) deaths. His sardonic intemperance tended to relate such obsession with physical decay to the way urban youth at play draws 'regenerative vigour from manure' in a world governed by a 'fimetic Providence'. ('Fimetic' is Ruskinian for shitty.) We are going to have to wait until Joyce's *Ulysses* before common human activities like pissing and shitting, menstruating and copulating, masturbating and nose picking, can be narrated without neurotic revulsion or smart satirical disengagement. Meanwhile, in a code easy for them to crack, Dickens rubs Victorian readers' noses in the difficulty of keeping things clean (and free of infection) in an excremental city crammed with suggestively filthy sites (from the manifest slum horrors of Tom-All-Alone's to the farcical avalanche of junk overwhelming poor Mr Jellyby when he opens a cupboard in his neglected household) and climaxing in the kind of fetid urban graveyard that Dickens in his humanitarian journalism recognises as the epicentre of contagion.

In such a fiction the heroes and heroines are those who humbly set out to put things in order, to clean things up. It may be only the good doctor Woodcourt trying to cleanse the bruised eye of a battered wife or Inspector Bucket determined to clear up the murder mystery (his apparently ludicrous name symbolising the unpretentious instrument of his would-be purifying act?). No wonder that the most conspicuous tragic victim is Jo, the devoted and harried crossing sweeper, or that my favourite fighter, too-young Charley, with her arms invariably covered in soapsuds, is supporting her family by 'doing' for the vile Smallweeds. It should not be missed, too, that Esther herself is purposefully nicknamed Dame Durden after the nursery-rhyme character who sweeps the sky. One of my most cherished wash-and-brush-up moments in the book (in lectures, I have read it out in full with relish) is that magnificent riposte by the rough brickmaker, 'all stained with clay and mud', to Mrs Pardiggle on her do-gooding mission to his damp, deprived and almost irremediably dirty home: 'Is this my daughter a-washin?' (She is "doing some kind of washing in very dirty water".) Yes, she is a-washin. Look at the water. Smell it! That's wot we drinks. How do you like it, and what do you think of gin, instead! An't my place dirty? yes, it is dirty – it's nat'rally dirty, and it's nat'rally unwholesome …'. Imagine Mrs Pardiggle to be an incompetent medical officer and we get an exemplary scene of the patient clamouring to be heard. Dickens provides us with Esther as the model of the good listener, even to a tirade that is in part the self-justification of a wife-abusing drunk, for here is the authentic indignation of the patronised, of someone unable to escape enslavement by dirt and disease. When GK Chesterton celebrated Robert Browning for composing the distinctively modern epic, since the poet had the gift of listening, more generously and inclusively, to the voices of the people, he might have said the same of Dickens, whose muck-raking epic is the convincingly and captivatingly polyphonic *Bleak House*.

Further reading

Ruskin J (1885) 'Fiction – Fair and Foul 1880–81' in *On The Road*.

17

Madame Bovary

by Gustave Flaubert

Charles Dickens' *Bleak House* ends with its heroine, Esther, celebrating the joys of being the wife of a country doctor. At more or less the same time (1851 onwards) another great writer, across the Channel in Rouen, was telling the story of a country doctor's wife who was not at all happy with either husband or lifestyle. Not happy? We male doctors ask ourselves: how is this possible? Who is this Gustave Flaubert and what does he know about the life of a country doctor's family? Let us investigate the author a little, before we open the book.

About the author

Now it so happens that when young Gustave was born in 1821, his father was director and chief surgeon of the municipal hospital in Rouen. The family actually lived in the hospital and little Gus and his sister would sometimes peep over the garden wall and watch their father doing autopsies. If he caught sight of them he would angrily wave them away with a bloody scalpel. I don't know if these childhood experiences affected Gustave at all, but at the age of 23 the young man began having nervous attacks with convulsions, hallucinations and unconsciousness. My informant is uncertain whether epilepsy was or was not confirmed. At any rate, he had to give up (gratefully) his training to be a lawyer. Instead he devoted himself to his writing. A year later, his father died from gangrene resulting from an abscess on the leg (remember that, because it will ring a bell later on). Gustave lived most of the rest of his life with his widowed mother, so don't tell me he didn't have plenty of time to hear about the downside of marriage to a doctor. He travelled a bit and he had a girlfriend (Louise Colet), but he complained that she disturbed his concentration. What he really wanted was to be left alone to get on with his writing. He was very serious about style and would spend hours revising a single sentence until it sounded perfect. And remember there were no word processors in those days. His subject was 'provincial life'. You might think he was fond of the country people in and around Rouen, but in fact he was rather superior and contemptuous of the *'petit bourgeois'* whom he regarded as either very naïve and stupid or absurdly pretentious. But when he created Emma, his heroine, he began to feel very deeply for her, and even identify with her (as we are about to do), although that didn't prevent him from treating her rather severely. The book was regarded as scandalous when it came out (in 1857) and it was actually the subject of an obscenity trial, just like *Lady Chatterley's Lover* nearly a century later. Like Lady Chatterley, Emma Bovary was acquitted, sales of the book took off and Flaubert became famous.

In the schoolroom

Now that we are eager to meet Emma, it is rather disconcerting to find that her entry on to the stage is delayed until Chapter 2. As the book opens we find ourselves in a classroom in a boys' school. The narrator appears to have been in the class himself and is recalling the scene from his childhood. A new boy is being introduced into the class of 15-year-olds. It is always difficult having to start a new school in the middle of term and this young man has no self-confidence whatever. He is tall and awkward with ill-fitting clothes and a very strange hat. To make matters worse, the teacher makes fun of him from the start and soon has all the kids laughing. Who is this unfortunate youth? His name is Charles Bovary, we are told, and his father was an army doctor who had to resign the service, tried business and farming, and failed at both. The story of young Charles is then told in flashback up to the point where he joins the class and embarks on a totally undistinguished school career. After three years (the narrator continues) 'he was taken away from school to study medicine'. The poor boy finds lectures on anatomy, physiology, pathology and so forth quite bewildering: 'he didn't understand a word of it; he couldn't grasp it however hard he listened'. Nevertheless he perseveres and 'to spare him expense, his mother sent him a little piece of baked veal each week by the carrier ...' (Flaubert is superb at supplying these important little details; he is particularly good on food). Poor Charles flunks his finals the first time but goes back, tries again and eventually qualifies as an 'Officer of Health', which I have to tell you was a slightly low form of medical life, not quite a proper doctor. He probably would not have reached MRCGP standard but, nevertheless, I think we should accept him as one of us.

Charles goes into general practice

As soon as he has his diploma his mother, who is quite a busy operator, finds a single-handed practice vacancy for him in a small town called Tostes. She also finds him a wife, a supposedly rich widow of 45, who is not just ugly but 'thin as a lath, with as many pimples as the spring has buds'. She proceeds to lay down the law about how he should live and then complains that he doesn't really love her. Oh dear, Charles, you great booby, why did you let this happen for goodness sake? And where will it end?

Chapter 2 opens, refreshingly, with a night call. All right, we don't like night calls, but at least it will get us out of that claustrophobic house. We are off on horseback, a journey of 18 miles across country to Les Bertaux, where a farmer, the good M Rouault, has broken his leg. As he rides along, Charles tries sleepily to remember all the different kinds of fractures and how to treat them (the way you do). Fortunately this fracture is a very simple one and farmer Rouault is a genial and grateful patient. Furthermore, his only companion is his daughter, Emma, who I guess must be about 18. Charles is immediately smitten. He is astonished at the whiteness of her nails. Her hands are otherwise unremarkable but, 'Her beauty was in her eyes – brown eyes, but made to look black by their dark lashes: eyes that came to meet yours openly, with a bold candour.' She also has black hair which sweeps round her head into a bun, leaving just the lobes of her ears visible. Her cheeks are like rosy apples. I think you get the picture. As the old man's fracture heals, Charles finds himself doing rather more return visits to the farm than is medically necessary. Even when the farmer is back on his feet (at 46 days) the doctor keeps turning up. Soon Charles's wife begins to notice and becomes jealous so that he has to promise not to go there any more. A little later his wife is swindled by her solicitor and she loses all her money. Charles's parents are furious, there are unseemly rows and then one day the unhappy first wife spits blood and conveniently dies.

What will happen now? Farmer Rouault comes to pay for his treatment (75 francs in 40-sou pieces and a turkey). The visits to the farm are renewed and Charles and Emma begin to see more of each other. One hot afternoon he finds her sewing in the kitchen. 'She had nothing round her neck and little drops of perspiration stood on her bare shoulders.' This is getting very erotic. They drink a glass of curaçao together and Emma tilts her head back, laughing as she tries to lick up the last few drops from the glass with the tip of her tongue. She takes him up to her room and shows him the little music books she won as school prizes. She chatters away and tells him all her likes and dislikes. That night he is unable to sleep for thoughts of Emma. For a long time he is too nervous to pop the question but finally he stammers to her father that he has something he wants to tell him. M Rouault has, of course, guessed what is going on between the two young people and has already decided that Charles will be a suitable son-in-law. So Charles and Emma get married and Emma becomes the second Madame Bovary (or the third if we count his mother as the first of the women who rule his life).

The wedding feast

The next chapter is a set-piece description of the wedding, the sort of thing at which Flaubert excels. We get a full picture of the guests, the horses, the procession, the clothes. This wedding is a really big affair, but as the families and their guests are 'provincial', Flaubert mocks their efforts at putting on the style unmercifully: 'And their shirts bulged out like breastplates! Heads were all freshly cropped, with ears sticking out and faces close-shaven. Some who had got up before it was light enough to shave properly showed diagonal slashes under the nose or cuts along the jaw as far across as a three-franc piece.' It's cruel but I'm afraid it is very funny. And as for the food, I can only give you a sniff of the goodies laid out in the cart-shed. 'On the table were four sirloins, six dishes of hashed chicken, some stewed veal, three legs of mutton, and in the middle a nice roast sucking-pig flanked by four pork sausages with sorrel. Flasks of brandy stood at the corners.' Don't you wish you had been there? Or perhaps you are a vegetarian? There are also dishes of wonderful wobbling custard 'with the initials of the newly-wedded couple traced on its smooth surface in arabesques of sugared almond'. After the lunch (which goes on till dusk) the party gets a bit riotous and a cousin has to be restrained by the bride's father from squirting water from his mouth through the key-hole of the happy couple's bedroom. Two days later Charles and Emma drive off back to Tostes and Charles's practice. There is a rather touching little passage in which the old farmer watches his now-married daughter departing with her husband and remembers his own wedding and his years of happiness with Emma's mother.

Married life

How will the Bovarys enjoy their married life? Charles thinks it's wonderful. He has endured years of misery and humiliation. In bed, his first wife's feet were like blocks of ice. 'But now, this pretty woman he adored was his for life. The universe for him was contracted to the silken compass of her petticoat.' He can't resist creeping up behind her and kissing the back of her neck. Well, some girls might rather enjoy that. Emma gives a little scream: but not, I'm afraid, of delight. Our bride is already feeling disenchanted with marriage and her groom. 'Before the wedding she had believed herself in love.' But where is the bliss, the passion and the ecstasy she was expecting?

It is time for a flashback to Emma's child and girlhood. At last Gustave allows us to enter into Emma's head and see the provincial world from behind those long dark eyelashes. And to feel part of her. We learn about her convent schooldays and her appetite for romantic novels, songs and coloured prints. This honeymoon period, she feels, should be the ecstatic fulfilment of all those adolescent yearnings. But stolid old Charles is not the lover of her teenage fantasies; 'his conversation was as flat as a street pavement on which everybody's ideas trudged past'. He can't swim, fence or fire a pistol. He's hopeless. Sadly, Emma is already bored with her new husband. She tries various ways of diverting herself from this crushing disappointment: she sketches, plays the piano; she even runs the house and manages the practice very efficiently. She tries to 'make herself in love' by reciting love poetry to Charles and singing to him in their garden by moonlight. Nothing happens. Finally, we sit with Emma in the garden as she pokes the grass irritably with her sunshade and repeats over and over: 'O God, O God, why did I get married?'

An excursion to a grand ball at a nearby chateau (including an overnight stay) raises her hopes of entering a more exciting social circle: she even has an intoxicating whirl round the dance floor with a *Vicomte*. But the invitation is not followed up and life for our heroine reverts to boredom and apathy. Her husband, blithely unaware of Emma's misery, is still contentedly enjoying his half of the marriage. Emma begins to decline and suffocate for lack of romantic oxygen. She gives up reading, drawing and playing the piano. She becomes anorexic. Charles, now seriously concerned, takes her to see his old consultant who diagnoses 'nervous trouble' and recommends a change of scene. Charles finds a new practice in a large market town and they prepare to depart. In the closing paragraphs of this electrically charged chapter, we watch apprehensively as Emma burns her wedding bouquet: 'The orange blossom was yellow with dust, the silver-trimmed satin ribbon frayed at the edges. She tossed it into the fire. It flared up like dry straw … The little cardboard berries popped, the wires twisted, the braid melted away and the shrivelled paper petals hovered like black butterflies at the back of the fireplace and finally vanished up the chimney.' And Flaubert follows up this vivid, shocking little cremation of Emma's honeymoon hopes with the last line of Part 1: 'When they left Tostes in March, Madame Bovary was pregnant.'

Part 2: life in Yonville

Flaubert takes us in to Charles and Emma's new home town before they arrive and gives us a conducted tour. As usual, it is the fine details in his descriptions which bring the place to life. Like this picture of the Yonville houses:

> *The thatched roofs, like fur caps pulled down over the eyes, hide nearly a third part of the low windows, which have thick bulging panes with a knot in the centre, like the bottom of a bottle. Against the plaster walls, diagonally crossed by black joists, leans an occasional sickly-looking pear tree, and in the doorway is a low swing gate to keep out the chicks that come to forage for brown bread-crumbs soaked in cider.*

Lucky little chicks! We carry on down the main street, observing the blacksmith's, the wheelwright's and the imposing notary's house. At last we reach the square in which we find the inn, the Golden Lion, and the chemist's shop (very important). We go into the inn and meet some of the local characters including the chemist himself, M Homais, 'a man in green leather slippers with a somewhat pock-marked face and a gold-tasselled velvet cap on his head. His face expressed nothing but self-satisfaction'.

Soon the little yellow local coach (L'Hirondelle) arrives with the Bovarys. They are late and somewhat dishevelled because Emma's pet greyhound had jumped out and run off. There is a very funny little paragraph about stories of the return of long-lost dogs, but you must find and relish that for yourselves. These details of life in Yonville are so delicious, I have to resist the temptation to quote more and more. I want to go there for a holiday and see it all for myself. But now we must attend to Charles and Emma, who are warming themselves in front of the fire at the Golden Lion. Emma's skin glows in the firelight and her trim figure catches the attention of a young student called Léon, of whom we shall hear more. Meanwhile, Charles is listening politely as Homais, the chemist, gives the new doctor a complete rundown on the history, geography, climate, epidemiology, etc., of Yonville. Well, any new GP needs to have a good relationship with the local pharmacist and Homais seems very ready to help in every way. However, it soon becomes plain that he is a tedious, pompous, loud-mouthed know-all. He brags about how well-informed he is about advances in medical practice and science generally. He clearly believes he could make a much better job of being the town doctor himself if he only had the diploma. We readers find him rather a joke, but he is also a little bit disturbing. Charles, of course, thinks he's wonderful and attends happily to all Homais's patronising advice.

So the Bovarys settle into Yonville and after a few months, Emma has her baby (a little girl). We are now hoping that things will improve for the young couple. Perhaps motherhood will suit Emma; or maybe Charles will buy her some flowers now and then or take her to another party. I am sorry to say, this is not what happens.

Emma and her lovers

Yes, Emma's unsatisfied romantic urges lead her, at first slowly and then with a rush, into adultery. They also lead her into debt, which, in the end, is even more serious. I will explain how this happens in due course; but first we must accompany our heroine (sorrowfully or excitedly, or perhaps both) down the primrose path of illicit love. The first suitor is young Léon, who observed her longingly in the Golden Lion when she arrived. They are introduced to each other and soon discover that they share an enthusiasm for music, poetry and romantic scenery. They have opportunities to meet socially because Léon lodges with the chemist and his wife; they even manage a long walk together by the river. By this time Léon is deeply in love with Emma but too shy to make a move. And she is not yet so deep in betrayal and rebellion as to encourage him. She remains virtuous: 'but within she was all desire and rage and hatred'. She dreams of eloping; she gets more irritable with Charles; she suffers nervous attacks of gasping and sobbing. Her maid remembers another woman who had a nervous illness which cleared up when she got married. '"But with me," replied Emma, "it didn't come on till I was married".'

After a while, Léon decides he can't stand the frustration any more and goes off to Paris, hoping to forget Madame Bovary. He is not long gone before lover number two comes on the scene in the shape of a suave, confident, 34-year-old landowner called Rodolphe Boulanger. Rodolphe calls in at the Bovary house because his servant is suffering from pins and needles and wants the doctor to bleed him. It's not clear whether Charles still believes in this sort of treatment, but when the patient is insistent one often gives in. During the bleeding, the basin is held by the chemist's apprentice, young Justine (who also nurses a hopeless, adolescent yearning for Emma). The sight of the blood makes him faint and he is revived by Emma, who spends some minutes untying his shirt strings with her dainty fingers (lucky lad). The way her yellow dress clings to her body as she bends down is acutely observed by M Rodolphe: 'Very nice,' he muses, 'Very nice, this doctor's wife! Pretty teeth, dark eyes, trim little foot, turned out like a Parisian.'

Unlike Léon, M Rodolphe is 'hard of heart and shrewd of head' and he knows exactly what to do. He decides he must have her. 'She would be tender, charming ... but how to get rid of her afterwards?' Well, that gives us an idea of what to expect from Rodolphe. It is very worrying (and, I'm afraid, arousing, for both Emma and her faithful readers). Soon, the doctor's wife and the smooth seducer are getting acquainted. Meanwhile the townsfolk are becoming aroused by the arrival of the grand Agricultural Show, which is being held in Yonville for the first time. There are displays of animals and produce, marching bands, prize-givings and endless speeches, all described by our author with loving irony. Emma and Rodolphe watch the show sitting together in the council chamber on the first floor of the Town Hall. Flaubert uses a brilliant, cinematic cross-cutting technique, switching rapidly between long shots of the public scene and intimate close-ups of Rodolphe flirting with Emma. Having made sure that she has fallen for him, Rodolphe then disappears for six weeks, leaving Emma to fret and pine. When he returns she falls helplessly into his clutches. He takes her riding (with Charles's encouragement, foolish man). Her horse has pink rosettes at its ears and a buckskin sidesaddle. They dismount in a clearing in the forest and by the side of a pond, they make love for the first time. Emma is really pleased with herself. 'I've a lover, I've a lover', she tells herself: at last she is just like one of the heroines in her storybooks. They begin secret assignations, at first at his place and then in the Bovary garden (or, if it's raining, in the consulting room) while Charles is out doing visits. But soon, Rodolphe begins to cool off and get bored with Emma. They continue their affair but Emma is aware that things are not the same. There is a touching little scene where she reads a letter from her kindly father, who thinks she is still happily married. She and Rodolphe will shortly part. But before they do, Flaubert inserts a bizarre little surgical episode which must grab our attention.

The operation for club foot

Homais the chemist, who keeps up to date with all the medical journals, has read about a new treatment for club foot. It so happens that the ostler at the Golden Lion, an old fellow called Hippolyte, has a club foot on which he stumps about quite happily. Homais thinks that if Charles were to correct the deformity using the latest method from Paris he could write it up for the papers and bring some fame and glory to the town. He tells Emma about the idea and together they urge Charles to have a go at it. This is like asking a GP who is only average at minor surgery to undertake a totally new procedure without even having seen one, let alone done one under supervision. But Charles agrees. He sends for the new treatise on Talipes and spends his evenings trying to work out the difference between varus, valgus and equinus. The patient is not at all keen to take part but Homais bullies him into it. Charles studies his foot dubiously: it is broad and horny with great thick toes: clearly it's an equinus, it even looks like a horse's hoof. And, come to think of it, even his name, Hippolyte, has a horsy sound. (It is curious the way horses keep cropping up in one form or another in this book; I expect someone has done a PhD on it.) But is it valgus or varus? With Homais in attendance and the whole town watching, Charles cuts through the Achilles tendon and encloses Hippolyte's lower leg in a special box he has constructed for the purpose. The same evening, Homais dashes off a description for the press: 'M Bovary, one of our most distinguished practitioners, operated on a clubfoot …'.

But five days later, the patient is writhing in terrible pain. The foot is infected and soon becomes gangrenous (you remember what happened to Flaubert's father?). When the gangrene rises to the knee, despite all their efforts, Charles has to send for a proper surgeon, the celebrated Carnivet of Neufchâtel. Carnivet is an unpleasant, arrogant fellow who sneers at them all and humiliates poor Charles: 'Straighten a clubfoot? – how can you straighten a clubfoot. You might as well try to straighten a hunch-back.' He proceeds to perform a mid-thigh amputation on the billiard table in the Golden Lion while the whole town listens to the wretched patient's agonised cries. As this is going on, Charles sits in his dining room staring at the fireplace. Emma watches him, full of disgust at his mediocrity. 'Perhaps it was valgus, then,' he says at one point. Poor chap, I feel really sorry for him and I have privately decided never to attempt any kind of minor surgery again.

I am sorry to say that Emma is not at all supportive. Angrily refusing his pathetic request for a kiss, she runs from the room, slamming the door so hard that the barometer falls to the floor. Soon she has plunged back into her affair with Rodolphe. But he is already thinking that it's time to end it. He agrees, halfheartedly to her eager plan for them to run away together. But when she waits for him to arrive on the appointed day, he sends his servant with a basket of apricots and letter telling her they must part (for her own good because society would be so cruel, etc.) and he himself will be leaving the country immediately for a long time.

Emma is distraught. She falls into another and more prolonged psychosomatic illness.

A night at the opera: the return of Léon

Emma's recovery is a slow one. She remains ill throughout the winter but begins to revive a little in the spring. Charles is persuaded to take her to Rouen to hear a famous tenor performing at the opera. The show is 'Lucia di Lammermoor,' and opera lovers will be quick to see that Donizetti's drama about a heroine who stabs the husband she doesn't love and then goes crazy, would appeal to Madame Bovary. In fact, the most exciting thing about the evening for Emma is the appearance in the audience of her old admirer Léon, who has been studying law in Rouen.

Their meeting at the opera house leads Emma into a second love affair. Léon is now a little more confident, while Emma has become experienced and reckless. They arrange to meet the next morning at the cathedral. This is an amusing scene in which their attempts to have a private passionate conversation are frustrated by the beadle who can't bear the idea of people looking round the church without the benefit of his rather extended guided tour. Outside the cathedral the lovers hail a cab and they embark on the famous *Madame Bovary* all-day ride in a cab with the blinds down. The driver is puzzled, the horses get exhausted; but inside the cab the lovers are at last united. Their subsequent meetings are more comfortably located. Emma persuades Charles to let her go to Rouen for three days to sort out his financial affairs following the death of his father. She and Léon have a delightful three-day 'honeymoon' in a nice hotel on the quayside. They take an evening boat trip and have dinner in a romantic little tavern. When she returns home she comes up with an ingenious way of seeing Léon regularly. She will tell Charles that she needs to go to Rouen every Thursday to have piano lessons. And so the affair continues. Emma is having a lovely time and I suppose we should be enjoying it with her; but where is it leading? How long will it be before Léon falls in love with someone his own age? And meanwhile another problem has been creeping up on our heroine: she is hopelessly in debt.

Emma's financial problems

Ever since her arrival in Yonville Emma has been carrying on another kind of 'affair' with an unscrupulous trader and money-lender called M Lheureux. The name suggests a purveyor of happiness (*heureux* is French for 'happy') and indeed M Lheureux aims to please his female customers by supplying fine clothes, linens, knick-knacks and fancy goods of all kinds at reasonable prices. And if a lady has a slight cash-flow problem, Lheureux is only too happy to arrange a little loan. At first Emma is contemptuous; but she soon needs money to finance her adventures with her lovers. She starts to sign bills of loan which, as soon as they fall due, are renewed by the obliging Lheureux. I find all this business about bills and notes of hand falling due rather difficult to follow: but it's quite clear that the more you borrow the more interest you have to pay and, if that is deferred too, you end up with a huge debt (just like with credit cards). To make matters worse, Charles has been borrowing from Lheureux as well because the practice finances have not been well-managed since Emma started having love affairs.

Things get worse and worse

On one of her return trips from seeing Léon, there is a sinister event which seems to foretell Emma's doom. The passengers in the coach (L'Hirondelle) are accosted by a hideous blind beggar with a horrible scabby face and a sightless leer. He runs after the carriage singing an obscene song, and when the coach stops in traffic (yes, traffic) he even thrusts his hat through the window for money. This spectre makes a number of appearances and seems to be a mocking nemesis figure for poor little Emma. After this episode, everything goes wrong. She gets cross with Léon, who seems to prefer having a long lunch with Homais to meeting her.

Then his family get to hear that he is carrying on with a married woman and he is advised to break it off to avoid scandal. Lheureux starts demanding his money back with menaces; Emma buys some time by selling off some cottages which Charles has inherited. But even that is not enough. Impatient for the return of his capital, Lheureux sends in the bailiffs and Emma has the agonising humiliation of seeing them draw up a list of her furniture for distraint. Unless she can raise 8000 francs in the next 24 hours the bailiffs will return and take everything – even Charles's medical equipment.

First she tries Léon, but he can't or won't help. Then she goes to the notary, a slimy fellow who takes her hand on to his knee and offers money only in return for sexual favours. Emma will not sink this low. In desperation, she rushes over to Rodolphe's magnificent country house. He is pleased to see her and quite willing to renew the affair but insists that he can't raise any cash. Emma unleashes a storm of bitter reproaches, flings one of his gold cufflinks against the wall (snapping the chain) and dashes back to Yonville. Now she is entering the chemist's house. Surely she won't try and borrow money from him? No, she is after something else. She encounters the terrified apprentice (who tragically still loves her) and demands the key to the laboratory where the poisons are kept. He refuses, but she knows where it is kept and takes it anyway. Before we can stop her, she is up there, seizing the blue jar and stuffing her mouth with arsenic powder.

The last days of the Bovarys

The last few chapters are almost unbearably sad and M Flaubert spares us none of the details. Charles tries frantically to revive his wife. He kneels sobbing by her bed and she says faintly: 'Don't cry … soon I shall be troubling you no more.' She tells him he is a good man, which indeed he is, but somehow it wasn't enough to be good. Two eminent consultants are summoned from Rouen and Paris but they can do nothing. Emma declines inexorably and dies. The last thing she hears is the mocking song of the malignant beggar from the street outside. The bereaved doctor is left to look after his little daughter, who is called Berthe and is now about six. I am afraid I have neglected her, but so has everybody else, especially her mother. Charles decides that at least he will look after her properly, even though they are now quite poor as a result of having to settle all Emma's debts. While Emma dies and Charles declines, Homais, the obnoxious pharmacist, continues to prosper. His journalism flourishes and he even writes a book (*A Statistical Survey of the County of Yonville*). He introduces all sorts of inventions and discoveries. His wife is proud of him and his children are all helping in the business. Charles dies suddenly in his garden, in the middle of a game with little Berthe. In the last line, Flaubert tells us with overwhelming irony that Homais 'has just been awarded the Legion of Honour'.

Some parting thoughts

I always feel very sad when I finish *Madame Bovary* and I think you will too. We have felt so close to her in everything she has gone through and now she is dead – while revolting people like Homais go blithely on with their self-satisfied lives. It is so unfair. If Gustave was alive, we should feel bound to ask him why? All right, he may have felt very superior to all these petty bourgeois people and merely wanted to observe their behaviour as if they were a colony of ants. But why, in that case, did he make us feel so tenderly about Emma? It is well known that when somebody did ask him questions like this he said; 'Madame Bovary, c'est moi!' I think while he was writing about her he must have discovered that he had begun to feel more in touch with her feelings (and some hidden ones of his own) than he had anticipated. Maybe the same thing happened to Tolstoy with Anna Karenin. Unhappily, there seems to have been a rule among nineteenth-century novelists that wayward heroines had to be terminated with extreme prejudice as an example to anyone who might think that adultery could be tolerated. We have to wait until 1922 before Molly Bloom is allowed to get away with it in *Ulysses*. But does Gustave have to dispose of his heroine with such relish and such grisly detail? Did he hate her as well as love her? We shall never know. But don't let the unhappy ending put you off. I urge you to make for Yonville as soon as possible; watch Charles happily eating his dinner after coming back from his rounds; let Emma pour out her discontents and cry on your shoulder; listen to Homais pontificating about the latest evidence-based medical discoveries; and watch those chicks enjoying their cider-soaked breadcrumbs.

The text

Madame Bovary (1857) by Gustave Flaubert. Translation by Alan Russell (1950) published by Penguin Books, London. Extracts reproduced by permission of Penguin Books Ltd.

18

The Rime of the Ancient Mariner

by Samuel Taylor Coleridge

Gillie Bolton

Beyond the shadow of the ship

The Ancient Mariner tells the tale of a voyage. It is the journey of his life, of yours and mine. Life as a journey is an old, tried-and-trusted metaphor. Homer started us off on it with his story of Odysseus's travels around the Aegean trying to get back from the Trojan Wars to his waiting wife Penelope, his home, son and throne.

The tale is presented as one told to an innocent audience: a *wedding guest*. This lad has to sit and listen to the grisly tale rather than sing and dance and drink at his friends' wedding. We are all the wedding guest, just as we are all the Ancient Mariner. The lad is told: stop, look, listen; don't just charge through life unheeding. Reflect upon its meaning to you, reflect upon where your actions might lead you or others.

Coleridge was a romantic poet. His message is: only once we have understood, accepted and made our peace with much about nature and life, can we begin to live it to the full – in harmony – only when we have learned:

> *He prayeth best, who loveth best*
> *All things both great and small.*

I'm rushing you on to the end here – this couplet concludes *The Rime of the Ancient Mariner*. But this story tells us no more than this: a life based on love, and an understanding that with love we can make anything happen, will be a life lived to the full. Eat your heart out ambition, avarice and desire for fame.

The story

Having started at the end, now I should go back to the beginning and fill you in on the narrative. It is a real ballad with plenty of story and is terribly easy to read – unputdownable even. It is written in simple language, and the magnificent rhythm and rhyme rolls you along with it – just like the sea journey it depicts.

The mariner's ship is taken by a storm down to the south of the southern hemisphere:

And through the drifts the snowy clifts
Did send a dismal sheen:
Nor shapes of men nor beasts we ken
The ice was all between.

The ice was here, the ice was there,
The ice was all around;
It cracked and growled, and roared and howled
Like noises in a swound.

Out of the blue, or perhaps I should say out of the white, an albatross appears. The crew hail it as a good omen – a live creature in the 'land of mist and snow'. It did bring them luck for: 'The ice did split with a thunder fit; / The helmsman steered us through! / And a good south wind sprung up behind.' But what did our hero, the mariner, do?:

With my cross-bow
I shot the albatross.

All seems tickety-boo at first as the ship continues to fly north, and it gets warmer. But the trouble is, it carries on getting warmer, and warmer:

> All in a hot and copper sky,
> The bloody sun at noon,
> Right up above the mast did stand,
> No bigger than the moon.
>
> Day after day, day after day,
> We stuck, nor breath nor motion;
> As idle as a painted ship
> upon a painted ocean.
>
> Water, water, everywhere,
> And all the boards did shrink;
> Water, water, everywhere,
> Nor any drop to drink.

What a use of words. The long 'o's in hot, copper, bloody, noon, moon; and then the two repetitions in the next stanza, and also in the last, hammer home to the reader the long deadly dreariness of it all. Not only is the ship hellish, but:

> The very deep did rot: Oh Christ!
> That ever this should be!
> Yea, slimy things did crawl with legs
> Upon the slimy sea ....
>
> And every tongue, through utter drought,
> Was withered at the root;
> We could not speak, no more than if
> We had been choked with soot.
>
> Ah well-a-day! What evil looks
> Had I from old and young!
> Instead of the cross, the albatross
> About my neck was hung.

There passed a weary time. Each throat
Was parched, and glazed each eye.
A weary time! A weary time!
How glazed each weary eye,
When looking westward, I beheld
A something in the sky.

Our hero bites his arm and sucks the blood to cry out at the sight of this ship. Of course they are in the doldrums where there is no wind, so this visitor is magically propelled. On it two horrific women – *Death* and *Life in Death* – are dicing for the crew's life. The former wins the majority, but the latter wins the mariner.

Coleridge likes to give us geographical information as we journey. He makes sure we know about the sun rising on the left as they travel south to the equator, and on the right as they journey northwards towards it. And he also tells us, in one of the delightful glosses which accompany the poem: 'No twilight within the courts of the Sun' (i.e. at the equator):

The sun's rim dips; the stars rush out:
At one stride comes the dark;

The short, jerky phrases here help with the sense of twilight being a rushed job compared with the glorious slow dance of light and colour associated with dusk and dawn nearer the poles. But Coleridge did not always get it right:

The hornèd moon, with one bright star
Within the nether tip.

It's a pretty image, but no star could ever get between the earth and the moon. I think Coleridge envisaged this impossible situation as being a bad omen, rather like the unknown author of the *Ballad of Sir Patrick Spens*[1] saw the image of the new moon with the old moon in her arms (when the dark side of the moon is visible beside the new crescent moon).

And the crew all die:

Fear at my heart as at a cup,
My life-blood seemed to sip! ...

One after one, by the star-dogged moon,
Too quick for groan or sigh,
Each turned his face with a ghastly pang,
And cursed me with his eye.

Four times fifty living men,
(And I heard nor sigh nor groan)
With heavy thump, a lifeless lump,
They dropped down one by one.

The souls did from their bodies fly, –
They fled to bliss or woe!
And every soul it passed me by,
Like the whizz of my CROSS-BOW! ...

Alone, alone, all, all alone,
Alone on a wide wide sea!
And never a saint took pity on
My soul in agony.

I hardly need to point out to you here the effect of the alliteration (repetition of consonants such as in thum**p**, lum**p**, and in a**ll**, a**l**one) and the assonance (repetition of vowels such as <u>a</u>ll and <u>a</u>lone), and the rhyme with 'woe' which brings us unremittingly to face what he did with his CROSS-BOW! Coleridge also used full internal rhyme to effect, as in: 'Instead of the cross, the Albatross ... '.

The mariner has a pretty bad time as you can imagine: 'And a thousand thousand slimy things / Lived on; and so did I. / ... I closed my lids, and kept them close, / And the balls like pulses beat; / For the sky and the sea, and the sea and the sky / Lay like a load on my weary eye, / And the dead were at my feet.' Full rhyme, alliteration, assonance and repetition are accompanied here by an extra-long line and an extra-long stanza.

The Ancient Mariner watches the soft motion of the moon (an image based on the memory of the moon clock face on Ottery St Mary church, where Coleridge spent his first years). Then, miraculously, he's watching beautiful water snakes, rather than 'slimy things':

Blue, glossy green, and velvet black,
They coiled and swam; and every track
Was a flash of golden fire.

Oh happy living things! no tongue
Their beauty might declare:
A spring of love gushed from my heart,
And I blessed them unaware …

The self-same moment I could pray;
And from my neck so free
The albatross fell off, and sank
Like lead into the sea.

And then it rains as he sleeps. The ship is driven home by the spirit. The curse which had remained in the eyes of the dead men is removed. But the mariner is still filled with dread, a dread we all recognise: 'Like one, that on a lonesome road / Doth walk in fear and dread / And having once turned round walks on, / And turns no more his head; / Because he knows, a fearful fiend / Doth close behind him tread.' I am reminded here of Wordsworth's similar dread when he stole a boat, and rowed across the lake at night,[2] in another poem I exhort you to read. The ship is propelled into harbour and the mariner is rescued by a hermit as it sinks.

We are returned to the present day with the mariner explaining to the wedding guest: 'Since then, at an uncertain hour, / That agony returns: / And till my ghastly tale is told, / This heart within me burns.'

Coleridge makes the mariner express what he himself had felt for many years, speaking of everyone's innate loneliness, especially those of us who know depression intimately:

O Wedding-Guest! this soul hath been
Alone on a wide wide sea:
So lonely 'twas, that God himself
Scarce seemèd there to be.

The mariner is doomed never to learn from his experience, but to travel seeking his next listener, to tell and retell, iterate and reiterate. His doom is never to move around the reflective learning cycle to build the knowledge gained into his understanding of himself and his life, and act more appropriately in the future. The audience (here the wedding guest and us) is doomed to miss out on a pleasurable life experience so that he can learn: going away 'A sadder and a wiser man'.

The mariner as a reflective practitioner

If the mariner were a medical or nursing reflective practice student of mine I'd really feel I'd failed.[3] What kinds of question could we encourage him to pursue which might help him towards this increase in understanding? It would certainly be about the moral and ethical implications of gratuitous killing. We could encourage him to explore his feelings about handling the ship beside the body of his dead brother's son (animated by a spirit) on the homeward journey. He could research the literature for the known consequences of destroying a bird of good omen.

I began this journey by telling you how the mariner *did* learn at the end about love being primary. The Duchess tells Alice in Wonderland: 'tis love, tis love which makes the world go round'. Alice remembers the Duchess earlier saying something quite different, and tartly says so: 'Somebody said that is done by everybody minding their own business!'[4] Well, if we all minded our own business we'd never learn from the actions of others, nor accept help in learning from our own experiences.

Coleridge presents us with this gloomy picture for the sake of literature. If the mariner had returned a happier and a wiser man, got married, raised children and grandchildren, we might never have heard the tale. Imagining ourselves a grandchild at his knee is not as romantic as being the chosen wedding guest. The mariner would lose his prophet status. We, the second tier of wedding guest, would not have been so spellbound. This despite us all liking a story to end happily ever after. Coleridge doesn't let us off the hook with: 'and he woke up to find himself comfortably in his own bed with the sun streaming in and the smell of fresh coffee drifting up from downstairs'. An incurable romantic, Coleridge would never have wanted his tragic mariner to achieve life satisfaction: how boring.

Coleridge as mariner

Coleridge is also saying something about himself, his own sense that he was forever in exile, forever having to travel onwards alone and leave behind. He was also a spellbinding talker, a vibrant dynamic figure in company, with an electrifying way of speaking. A scholar of Greek and Latin literature he was extremely well-read and knowledgeable as well as being brilliant in argument. When in company he had to shine in conversation and fix his listener with his 'glittering eye'.

Furthermore, 'part of Coleridge's genius was for wholly disrupting the lives and expectations of most of those who came in close contact with him'[5], particularly young men who were drawn to him, dazzled by his magnetism: listening to him 'like a three years' child' (and then sadly inexorably bitterly disappointed in him). The late eighteenth century, early nineteenth was a period of respect for fraternal feelings: the Age of Sensibility.

Coleridge did also exalt sisterly love, always regretting the early death of his beloved sister, Nancy. Dorothy Wordsworth's devotion to her brother William was one of her attractions to Coleridge. He was also wildly profligately sexual in his early years. But then his first love married another, his relationship with his wife Sara did not last long, and he spent his later life in hopeless love for another Sara, whom he called Asra. It's interesting to note there are no women in *The Ancient Mariner*, unless you count the horrific spectre of hags dicing on the death ship.

The Ancient Mariner was written when Coleridge was young. Towards the end of his life, he was uprooted, unsettled, had been separated from Sara for many years, was estranged from his beloved son Hartley (who followed his father in being unreliable), hopelessly in love with another Sara with whom he couldn't have a relationship, and heavily addicted to opium. Both his health and his writing suffered, and he died prematurely of heart disease. *The Ancient Mariner*, a story of loss and wandering, good and bad omens not quite fulfilled, must itself have seemed like a bad foretelling.

A bit of biography

Coleridge was the youngest of ten children, most of whom were very successful. Coleridge's father, who was also successful, died when he was eight. He was sent away to an extremely abusive boarding school from whence he returned rarely. 'He developed the self-portrait of a precocious highly imaginative child, driven into "exile" in the world, before he was emotionally prepared for its rigours ... He was to be a solitary voyager, an archetypal "son of the earth", an orphan of the storm, flung out to wander over the world in search of visions. Or so, most wonderfully, he said.'[6]

Another poet who was blighted by the premature death of her father when she was eight was Sylvia Plath. She also never recovered from this loss, and never forgave him. He is the subject of some of her most vivid last poems.[7]

The pre-exile child, Sam, was a dreamer. From a very young age he read obsessively. The *Arabian Nights* introduced him to the story structure, to the notion of a quest and to the fantasy that there are powerful forces at work upon our lives.

Coleridge's Cambridge undergraduate years were marked by his passion for *pantisocracy*. He and others planned to move to the banks of the Susquehanna where they would live in fraternity, equality and harmony with nature. Remember, this was a heady period of anti-slave trade and of the early French Revolution, when all thinkers worth anything were desperate to be in France, or at least doing something towards 'The Cause'. His sense of fraternity extended to animals. Later, when writing *The Ancient Mariner* at Nether Stowey, he was torn about killing the mice which tormented them: the mice seemed almost as important to him as an albatross.

His undergraduate career was wild and profligate. To escape the shame of this, and his debts, he enlisted as a volunteer private in the 15th Light Dragoons, as Silas Tomkyn Comberbache. He couldn't ride, and with a bottom covered in boils, he was detailed to care for a fellow-dragoon with smallpox, in the 'pest house'. For eight days and nights he did not undress, but bathed and fed his comrade through the fever. This exposure to extreme sickness and hallucination probably gave him material for *The Ancient Mariner*.

During these years Coleridge and friends went on many energetic walking holidays, communing with nature. He later said that finding unexpected water under a stone on the summit of Penmaenmawr when lost with a friend, benighted and fearful they were pursued by monsters, affected his depiction of the mariner.

He was a very enthusiastic young man. His many, many letters are punctuated liberally with exclamation marks, as is *The Ancient Mariner*.

The Rime of the Ancient Mariner was composed while Coleridge lived in Nether Stowey, Somerset, with his wife Sara and baby son, Hartley: a time of unusual peace and domestic happiness. He had recently given up his degree, his pantisocratic plans and other ideas such as the law.

He had encouraged William Wordsworth and his sister Dorothy to live nearby and they spent many, many hours walking many, many miles both by day and night, talking metaphysics and poetry, and observing nature. So much so that they were suspected of being spies (their political sympathies with the Jacobins were well known), and were spied upon themselves as they walked and talked and wrote poetry.

Writing, rewriting and publication

The Ancient Mariner took five months to compose, during which time Coleridge also wrote *Kubla Khan* and *Frost at Midnight*. Completely different from each other, these celebrate two sides of Coleridge. *Kubla Khan* was occasioned by a medicinal dose of opium while resting at a remote farmhouse on a coastal walk nearby. It gives a fantastical magical land (very much an opium fantasy with huge magnificent structures). It was never finished, mostly because Coleridge's opium reverie was interrupted by a 'person from Porlock'. It seems he hoped to return to it for many years, but was unable to. Its fragmentary nature, however, is one of its charms.

Frost at Midnight offers a peaceful domestic picture in the cottage with frost outside, fire inside and sleeping baby. He refers to an aspect also vital to the Ancient Mariner: the healing, nurturing power of nature. Coleridge believed in the 'child of nature', that children should be nurtured and taught by nature, and that adults could easily mess this up. If I've enthused you with the *Mariner*, please also read these other two magnificent poems (much shorter than the *Mariner*).

The ballad includes many of Coleridge's deepest philosophic concerns, themes of exile and homecoming, the problematic nature of the relationship between people and nature, his psychological fascination with states of madness, dreams and hallucination which exist in the midst of the waking world (remember it was written a hundred years before Freud's great works). Coleridge explored the origins of evil and the sense of guilt and spiritual anxiety which he always felt. He was a Unitarian lay preacher with strong beliefs and sense of the power of evil, despite the growing fashion for atheism among those with revolutionary sympathies. He explored the effect of mankind's impious impact on nature, in the killing of the albatross. This seems particularly apposite to us now, with global warming, BSE, and foot and mouth obsessing us.

Just before writing this ballad, an unstable young man came to stay with the Coleridges. He was a fervent admirer of Coleridge and had prevailed upon his rich father to pay Coleridge as his tutor. Being with Coleridge much excited him, and Coleridge had to nurse him exhaustingly through a long series of epileptic fits and delirium. More material not only for the fantasy scenes of the mariner, but also for the role of the wedding guest.

Coleridge had never travelled at this early stage, but a *History of Greenland* by Crantz gave him images of desolate icy wastes, a giant bird and a powerful good spirit. We don't know about the influence of opium upon this work, but he did say that parts of *The Ancient Mariner* were written from somewhere outside his conscious control. And it reads like a visionary work.

The Rime of the Ancient Mariner was first published anonymously in a volume of *The Lyrical Ballads* (1798) with poems by Wordsworth. It was badly received, particularly by the poet Southey who reviewed the volume. Wordsworth felt that *The Mariner* put potential buyers off with its ghastly images. Coleridge told him that the publishers had said that lots of copies had been sold to seafaring men who took a professional interest in the mariner's journey. Whether this was true or not, we do know that many contemporary readers made little sense of it. Of course the sense it makes to us over 200 years later is partly due to the way Coleridge's writing, and that of the other romantics, have deeply affected understandings of ourselves, our lives and our roles in the world.

Once readers, such as Byron for example, had become much more used to the Romantic tradition, *The Ancient Mariner* became popular. This was the period of the gothic novel (as parodied by Jane Austen in *Northanger Abbey*), which reached its height in Mary Shelley's *Frankenstein* (written, believe it or not, when she was 19) (another must-read).

Coleridge altered and added to *The Ancient Mariner* on a voyage to the Mediterranean on an armed merchant ship, the *Speedwell*, running away from family and commitments, taking with him new boots, a sunhat and a pair of green solar spectacles, and leaving his children a game of spillikins. He also, much later, wrote the gloss that appears alongside the stanzas in the voice of a learned antiquarian – a seventeenth-century Christian commentator seeking to interpret the ballad like some mystical allegory of punishment and redemption.

Classical influences

Coleridge was widely read in classical as well as contemporary literature. *The Ancient Mariner* is part of a time-honoured genre of adventure, quest, rite of passage poems and stories: Beowulf, Odyssey, Nordic Sagas, aboriginal dreamtime cycles, Startrek, Mallory's *Morte d'Arthur*, Boccaccio, Chaucer's *Canterbury Tales*, Milton's *Paradise Lost*, Dante's *The Divine Comedy*, the ancient Bablylonian epic of *Gilgamesh, The Hitchhikers' Guide to the Galaxy* to name but a few. In a way, the rite of passage which is being undergone in *The Ancient Mariner* is that of life itself – life as a preparation for death, for whatever comes next. Or perhaps it's a rite of passage for life itself.

The ancient Greek playwrights Sophocles, Aeschylus and Euripedes present a powerful notion of fate, and the involvement of the gods in our lives. They paint a picture in which human actions inevitably lead to divine, fateful reactions. For example, when Orestes (*The Oresteia* by Aeschylus) kills his mother, he is inevitably pursued by the Furies because he has offended against the laws of the gods (nature). This even though Orestes was avenging the bloody death of his father at the hands of his mother Clytaemnestra. He is only saved by divine intervention, when Athene takes the tormented young man off the hook of fate.

The Ancient Mariner is saved when he is given the gift of perceiving the 'slimy things' as 'happy living things' – beautiful water snakes – which he blesses 'unaware'. He is saved again when the spirit with 'a softer voice, / As soft as honeydew' maintains 'The man hath penance done, / And penance more will do.' Not quite the voice of Athene, who was a warrior goddess, but still divine intervention.

The gods play with us, but they do play with us according to their own laws. We get our comeuppance. Medea (Euripides) deserves the misery of Jason's betrayal of her because of the bloody deeds she undertook to secure him when she first met him; and he deserves that she horrifically kill their sons, his new wife and father-in-law. Only the gods can stop the chain of punishment, with redemption. Antigone (Sophocles) sins against human law and willingly loses her life, but redeems the sin of her father, Oedipus, by her noble deed in keeping with the laws of the gods. (More books for you to read, if you haven't.) Of course these themes are taken up in Coleridge's own fervently held religion: the Bible is a story of blood, love and redemption.

Endnote

We seem to have covered a magnificent trajectory, helmed by Coleridge. I am writing this on a gloriously sunny, bitterly cold, pair of days, travelling by train from Derbyshire's Hope Valley where I live, to Coleridge's Somerset. My journey has been much befouled by Virgin Trains' muddles and confusions, and my voyage is towards working with a group of Masters' students on reflective practice. The Hope Valley is not quite the Romantics' Lake District, but it is pretty magnificent, dour and magical, particularly in the present snow. I am returning to work with a group of medical undergraduates on medicine and literature (one of whom gave us a magnificent introduction to Keats's *Ode on a Grecian Urn*). A chance and delightfully romantic congruence.

I'm going to leave you at Hope Station (two stops after mine on the Hope Valley Line) with a suggestion. Write the story of a journey of your own, a dream voyage, an allegorical trip. Invent a character, and places, and a form of transport (send it to me). And see where you end up. Down a rabbit hole, on the shores of Ithaca, back in your own bed with your cocoa still hot?

References

1   Anon, The Ballad of Sir Patrick Spens. In: J Wain (ed) (1986) *The Oxford Library of British Poetry*, vol 1, p 39. Oxford University Press, Oxford.

2   Wordsworth W (edn of 1985) The Prelude. In: J Wordsworth (ed) *Selected Poems*, pp 41–76. Cambridge University Press.

3   Bolton G (2001) *Reflective Practice: writing and professional development*. Sage, London.

4   Carroll L (1865(1954)) *Alice in Wonderland*. JM Dent, London, p 76.

5   Holmes R (1989) *Coleridge: early visions*. Penguin, London, p 142.

6   Holmes R (1989) *Coleridge: early visions*. Penguin, London, pp 1–2.

7   Plath S (1965) *Ariel*. Faber & Faber, London.

19

Serving suggestions for teachers

In this final chapter, I would like to consider some of the ways in which our selection of classic books might be used in teaching. A number of medical schools in the UK have begun to include literature seminars in their medical school curriculum as part of a medical humanities course.[1,2] A few general practice vocational training schemes have also included sessions on general reading on a regular or an occasional basis.[3] Similar courses have been widely used in US medical schools for many years.[4,5]

Most of the texts used in literature courses for medical students have been selected because they illustrate very directly the kind of experiences which doctors and patients have to go through and the moral dilemmas they may find themselves in. Examples which address the doctor's problems and choices are William Carlos Williams's *The Use of Force*, AJ Cronin's *The Citadel* and those parts of *Middlemarch* by George Eliot which deal with the difficulties of Dr Tertius Lydgate.

The patient's point of view is well represented in Tolstoy's *The Death of Ivan Illytch*. Medicine and literature courses may also use books and short stories which are not literary classics and not even examples of the best writing; but they do focus on important themes which the teacher wants the students to think about and discuss.

The texts in this book, on the other hand, have been chosen because they are outstanding works of literature. They are also particular favourites of ours, which means that we can write about them from the heart. Some have principal characters who are doctors and, in a number of others, doctors seem to have crept in and found minor roles for themselves. Charles Bovary, the doctor husband of Flaubert's Madame Bovary, makes readers think about the problems of being a doctor from time to time, but these are incidental. His main purpose is to be a decent, kindly man who, unhappily, fails to understand where his wife is coming from. Tertius Lydgate, in *Middlemarch*, gets a good deal of coverage in his medical role from George Eliot, but his problems are only partly to do with his profession and we are just as interested in all the other narrative threads and moral questions which make up a work of extraordinary richness.

So the aims of a learning programme based on these texts might be as follows:

- To learn how medicine and literature connect with one another.

- To realise that a close reading of a text can be as revealing as a close study of a patient.

- To gain pleasure and spiritual refreshment from reading and learning about some of the best books ever written.

- To be touched and changed by the emotional impact of great writing about human beings.

- To make some of this writing a permanent part of one's inner world.

We need to bear in mind that there may be different responses from groups at different ages and stages. Students may come to the text being studied completely new – or they may have read it in school. They will be looking at doctor–patient encounters with a fresh eye, and will be particularly aware of the attitudes and behaviours of their consultant teachers. GP registrars will have begun to struggle with the difficulties of tuning in to 'difficult' characters in the surgery and will enjoy being able to warm to fictional characters as human beings.

More senior doctors will, I hope, simply enjoy the chance to revisit old favourites or, at last, to be able to read books which they have always respected but found too difficult.

Now to the practicalities. How can our chosen texts, some of them very long, be incorporated in a limited number of seminars? I will offer a number of different methods, each appropriate for a particular work. All the methods (except one) involve small group work and are best suited to a class of between nine and 12 people.

Indian Camp by Ernest Hemingway

In Chapter 8, Brian Glasser has already demonstrated how he uses this amazing story in seminars for medical students. The story is short enough to be read when the students arrive. After eliciting their initial reactions, Brian then divides them up into small groups of two or three and gives each group a theme to work on, asking them to support their conclusions with material from the text. The groups then report back and there is a general discussion. Sometimes the tutor then introduces other texts, literary or medical, for comparison. Readers are referred back to Chapter 8 for a full account of this method.

A Country Doctor by Franz Kafka

I was particularly keen to introduce students and GP registrars to this story and I happily adopted (and adapted) Brian's technique. The story is another very short one (only six pages), but its surreal style makes it more difficult to grasp at a single reading. So I circulate copies to the group a few days before and ask them to read it before they arrive.

I then divide them into three groups and give each group a different task. Group one are asked to plot the course of the story, divide it into its various phases and say what they think is happening at each stage. I also ask them to look at the way the story is written and how this enables its effects to be achieved.

The second group's assignment is to think about what the story has to say to doctors. (There is plenty of material here about night visits, demanding patients, angry doctors, dissembling about a fatal diagnosis and professional 'burnout'.) Group three are slightly stunned when they find that their job is to find out as much as they can about Kafka's life and personality. They are provided with a serious biography and several copies of an excellent comic strip biography.[6]

After about half an hour, I bring the groups together and ask them to feed back their findings. Usually I ask the biographical group to go first. Brian Glasser has written (in Chapter 8) about the intense curiosity we feel about the personal lives of the authors of our favourite books. We feel (quite rightly in my view) that the author must have poured himself into the book (or at least drawn up a few bucketfuls from the depths of his unconscious). We want to know more about him (or her) and we are sure that this knowledge will help us to understand the book better. As Brian says, this approach is now deeply unfashionable in academic circles, where successive movements – structuralism, deconstructionism, postmodernism – whose names I can barely differentiate, let alone understand, have ruled that we should concentrate on the text and ignore the author. I think there is an analogy with medicine here. It seems to me that the modern critics are like the stricter proponents of evidence-based medicine, who base their conclusions on the texts of trials and meta-analyses. Those of us who want to know what sort of person the author was are more like the doctor who wants to know about the person who has produced the clinical narrative of symptoms and signs. With literature, as in medicine, there is much to be said for a combined approach and it is always worth looking at the way a writer achieves his or her effects by the use of symbolism, imagery and different narrative styles.

This digression (for which I apologise) began with the group who have been learning about Kafka's life. It is amazing how quickly they can piece together the strange story of the genius of Prague. And once they have heard it, it doesn't take long for all three groups to realise that there is a lot of Kafka and his personal preoccupations in *A Country Doctor*. For a discussion of what these are I will refer you back to Chapter 2. I think it is worth reminding the group that, although Franz Kafka emerges as a very strange bloke, we remember him and read his books because he was also a uniquely gifted writer.

I have 'done' *A Country Doctor* with groups of students, GP registrars and (in the USA) a group of family medicine department faculty. I have neglected, so far, to do any proper evaluation but it seems to be well received. Most of the participants start off knowing nothing about Kafka so they are launched on a steep learning curve. I hope that some of them go on to read more of his stories and novels.

I have also used the same method with a different Kafka story: *The Metamorphosis.* This, you may remember, is the one about the man who wakes up after troubled dreams to find that he has turned into a beetle. This story (a little longer at about 50 pages) is rich in medical metaphors although a doctor is only briefly mentioned.

Anna Karenin by Lev Tolstoy

Now we must consider how to deal with full-length novels. Clearly it would be expecting too much to ask medical students or registrars to read the whole of a 900-page book before coming to the class. The choice seems to lie between setting selected extracts from the book or asking people to read the opening section: anything from a chapter to a hundred or so pages. With *Anna Karenin,* my suggestion would be for everyone to read Part 1, which consists of 34 chapters and about 150 pages. This would have been the first instalment, published in a monthly magazine, a year before the book appeared as a whole. In this first section, we are introduced to the unfaithful but likeable Steve Oblonsky and his family; we get to know Levin and experience with him his meeting with Kitty at the skating rink and his first, unsuccessful, proposal. Anna will shortly arrive in Moscow from St Petersburg and encounter Vronsky at the railway station. We go to the ball and share Kitty's pain as she watches Vronsky and Anna, totally absorbed in each other. Levin goes sadly home to the country;

Vronsky and Anna meet again on a train journey; Anna returns to her husband and son; and finally Vronsky slips back into his life as a young, single officer. But we know that life will not be the same now for either of them.

When the session starts, I would try to establish how much everybody has read and with how much enjoyment. What is the significance of the famous first sentence? Who has read it before? Was it as they remembered it? What are their initial impressions of the main characters? I find it useful, with the help of the group, to construct a genogram or family tree showing the relationship of the Oblonsky and Shcherbatsky families. We might also discuss the personalities of the chief characters, the most memorable scenes and the way the book is written and constructed. As in the previous examples, much of this exploration can be done in small groups followed by a plenary session. If the session goes well, at least some of the class will want to go on reading and finish the book. There is not much of strictly medical interest in this first instalment: my main hope is that the students will begin to appreciate the miraculous way in which Tolstoy breathes life into his characters and makes us feel with them and for them. If they can transfer some of the empathy and compassion they have experienced to their relationships with patients, then so much the better.

Ulysses by James Joyce

With this book, I would suggest a sampling approach rather than a sequential reading of the first hundred pages. As my essay indicates, it is not necessary, perhaps not even desirable, for a first-time reader to follow the chapters in numerical order – and anyway they don't have numbers. The class could start by reading a brief overview of the novel and its structure (Chapter 7 of this book might serve for this purpose). Then they could study a few selected chapters. I would begin with Telemachus (Chapter 1), because one should know how books begin and because the interplay between Stephen and Buck Mulligan is not too difficult to follow. Then cut to Calypso (Chapter 4) to introduce Bloom and the stream of conscious narrative at its most endearing.

Those two are essential: you could then add one or two or three more depending on your estimate of the students' enthusiasm. Lestrygonians (Chapter 8) stays with Bloom and the streets of Dublin and is all about food. In Cyclops (Chapter 12), Joyce uses a different (unreliable) narrator with some interpolated parodies. He also shows Bloom stoutly defending his liberal beliefs before taking flight from a hail of anti-Semitic abuse. Then you might be daring and get them to read a little of Chapter 15 (Circe, the brothel-dream sequence) and finish up with a few pages from Molly Bloom's monologue (Chapter 18 and last, Penelope).

If this is too much, an alternative would be to read only Telemachus and Calypso as complete chapters and supply brief extracts from the others so that the students can catch something of the different flavours of Joycean style. It might be interesting to discuss how everybody reacts to 'modernist' ways of telling a story in different voices, which can be disconcerting when first encountered. Patients also tell their stories in a variety of narrative styles, which can be confusing and irritating. As with literature, a little patience and perseverance on the part of the 'reader' can be very rewarding.

For the small group work, each group could be asked to focus on a different chapter. The whole class could then read or listen to some of the extracts. (Does anyone do a good Dublin accent?) The session could conclude with a discussion about the book as a whole. I do hope they will keep reading it. Perhaps, years later, some of them will become dedicated Joyceans.

Tess of the d'Urbervilles by Thomas Hardy

Many students and registrars will be familiar with this one already. It is straightforward to read and so I recommend that you ask your class to read the whole thing over the summer holidays. Small groups could discuss different themes, such as Hardy's treatment of nature and the rural life; the character of Tess, and Hardy's treatment of her; and attitudes to female sexuality (have they changed?). The discussion might be better if each person knows in advance which theme his or her group will be addressing.

Some members could be asked to find out about Hardy's life and times and it would be interesting to see how many other Hardy books people have read.

A Midsummer Night's Dream by William Shakespeare

There is really no alternative but to take them to see the play. If this one is not available, then almost any Shakespeare play currently being performed in your area will do. You will discover that some of your flock have never seen a live performance of a Shakespeare play in their lives so the experience will be a revelation. But the language is a little difficult to follow at first and some knowledge of the plot can be very helpful. For *A Midsummer Night's Dream*, Chapter 3 can be circulated to everybody to read before you go to the theatre. For other plays I suggest that you get hold of a copy of the text and write your own.

Stories partly about doctors

These include *Middlemarch* and *Madame Bovary*. I recommend that you resist any temptation to extract the doctors and serve them up to your students without their proper context. *Middlemarch* is often cited as a novel which has much to say about the vocation of medicine and there is a limited truth in this. But to look only at Lydgate would be to deprive readers of the company of Dorothea and Mary Garth and all the other characters. There is much more to learn about human beings and their feelings from a study of the novel as a whole. By all means allow one small group to discuss Lydgate and the doctor's conscience, but make sure that Dorothea and Casaubon are there as well.

And finally ...

One or other of the methods outlined above should be suitable for all the other texts described in this book. Of course you can design your own variations or do something entirely different. The main thing is to present the books to your students in a way which invites their participation and challenges them a little without intimidating them or making them feel that they are out of their depth or have wandered into the wrong class. It is advisable not to talk too much or dazzle the class with your own interpretations. Mention a few of your favourite bits by all means, but offer them sparingly. It is much better if the seminar members develop their own relationship with the book and read extracts which appeal to them personally. If possible, everyone should have their own copy of the book being discussed. Classic texts are very reasonably priced these days and if modest funds are available, I recommend buying everybody a paperback copy of *Anna Karenin* or whatever book you decide to study. The gift of a book makes everyone feel valued. They will be able to write notes in the margins. If the class has been enjoyable they will treasure the books. And keep reading them.

References

1   Downie RS, Hendry RA, Macnaughten RJ, Smith BH (1997) Humanising medicine: a special study module. *Medical Education.* **31**: 276–80.

2   Clews G (2000) Literature in medicine: a novel approach. *BMA News Review.* **12 August**: 22–6.

3   Salinsky J (1990) Can reading novels make me a better doctor? English literature in the half-day release course. *Postgraduate Education for General Practice.* **1**: 18–22.

4   Hunter KM, Charon R, Coulehan JL (1995) The study of literature in medical education. *Academic Medicine.* **70**: 787–94.

5   Squier H (1998) Teaching humanities in the undergraduate medical curriculum. In: T Greehalgh, B Hurwitz (eds) *Narrative Based Medicine.* BMJ Books, London.

6   Mairowitz DZ, Crumb R (1993) *Kafka for Beginners.* Icon Books, Cambridge.

Index